ISIZULU

ISIZULU

A Manual For Health Care Workers

Mthunzi Thusi

Speaking IsiZulu in the Clinical Context

This book was printed in the United States of America.

To order additional copies of this book, contact:
Xlibris Corporation
0-800-644-6988
www.xlibrispublishing.co.uk
Orders@xlibrispublishing.co.uk
300968

CONTENTS

INTRODUCTION

S OUTH AFRICA IS a diverse country, this not only applies in terms of race but language and culture as well. After the democratic elections in 1994; eleven languages were put forward as officially acceptable mediums of exchanging information, and these have different popularities and are often regional (geographical prominence) in nature. The four most popular languages are isiZulu, isi Xhosa, Afrikaans and English in that order. English is the medium of instruction; it is used in most institutions for teaching and learning purposes; more than 80% of the time.

Basic knowledge of other languages for health care practitioners therefore becomes an important skill. Attempts have been made to address this matter and variable results have been yield; poor follow up has been made. This manual has been designed to equip health care practitioners with an adequate grip of English (basically all of them) to attain a level of competence in history taking and conducting an examination in one of the popular official languages, isiZulu. The manual has been designed such that it can be put to use by practitioners with some basics to increase their use and extend it to other aspects of patient interaction and those that need to start-up with the basics.

The author deems it important to mention that isiZulu as a language is broad; the manner of use depicted in this manual is general and basic. Like all other languages more is covered via interaction, speaking to people and learning more which is regrettably not covered by the manual. With adequate integration into daily use the aspects covered by the manual can be mastered within a matter of weeks and this gives assurance on fundamentals of use of the language in the patient interaction situation.

I trust that whosoever gets to use the manual relishes it and takes pride in speaking.

THE CULTURE

THE ISIZULU CULTURE has gone through a lot of refurbishing, it has been affected by the cataclysm of migrant labour, the changing education systems, the dynamics in living arrangements and people moving to towns wherein there are coexisting languages. There are regional variations in the language in the new South Africa, the admixture with other languages has been unavoidable and subtle styles of speaking exist in different regions. This manual plans to give an acceptable standard of the language that shall span through across various levels of comprehension.

The isiZulu speaking nation is a respectful and modest group of individuals, but this may come across as out of the truth to most that have had interactions with them but unanimously all will agree that they are a generous group of individuals even though there is usually very little to offer. The respect for the older is one crucial value and hallmark of the indigenous African nations of South Africa and the Zulu nation is no exception. The social fiber and the spirit of "ubuntu" have been put into question; debates about these have been topical of late however these are issues that are beyond the ambit of this manual.

The author hopes for this particular manual to open gates for other languages to have a backbone, Braille and the route to follow to come to the fore as South Africa is mosaic and this needs to reflect.

ACKNOWLEDGEMENTS

THE AUTHOR WOULD like to extend a word of appreciation to the following individuals viz: Marcus Mathale, Lwazi Mjiyako, Zamalotshwa Thusi, Prof. D. Prozesky and Zubair Randeree in no particular order for the invaluable contribution they made to the realization of this work.

May God bless their source of patience and ensure that it ever and overflows with the kind they showed to me.

THE LANGUAGE

I SIZULU AS A language is not different from others, words are put into use; they come in all forms (nouns, pronouns, verbs, adjectives etc.), information is conveyed in different forms (positive and negative statements, commands, information, requests etc,), there are tenses that are used (present, past, future etc.) and sentences are constructed in a particular way.

The language has been growing and moving with the times but some words are not primitively from the language i.e. they are derived; for some this is apparent for others it is not so obvious; an example, of a simple derivation a machine is "umshini" in isiZulu and that of a not so obvious one is television which is "umabonakude."

In the next section of the manual the building blocks of the isiZulu language shall be looked closely into and put into use for better comprehension.

NOUNS—AMABIZO

THERE ARE SIXTEEN classes of nouns, all nouns that one would come across in their use of the language falls into one of the classes. In general the nouns in their singular form fall into the odd numbered category, and the subsequent even number is the noun in its plural form. Below are the classes of nouns and an example of a noun has been given in each case.

CLASSESS OF NOUNS—IZIGABA ZAMABIZO

   1. Um(u)—   **umu**ntu   (person)

Other nouns in this class—umufi (the deceased), umfelokazi (A widow), umlungu (a white person), nouns in this class of nouns usually depict a person.

   1a. U—   **u**fezela   (scorpion)

Other nouns in this class—ugogo (grandmother), u-Johaness (a person's name), ubhejane (a rhinoceros); nouns in this class describe animals in singular form, are used to refer to a person as a third person etc

   2. Aba-/Abe—   **aba**ntu   (people)

Other nouns in this class—abelungu (white people), abafelokazi (widows), abathakathi (witches); plural form of nouns in class1.

2a. O—   **o**fezela   (scorpions)

Other nouns in this class—ogogo (grandmothers), o-Johaness, obhejane (rhinoes); plural form of nouns in class 1a.

3. Umu—   **umu**thi   (medicine/tree)

Other nouns in this class—umqamelo (a pillow), umlomo (mouth), umuzi (a house), describe things that are tangible

4. Imi—   **imi**thi   (medicines/trees)

Other nouns in this class—imiqamelo (pillows), imilomo (mouths), imizi (houses); plural form of nouns in class 3.

5. I—   ikhanda   (head)

Other nouns in this class—ikhabe (a watermelon), iqolo (the back), ijazi (a jacket); describe body parts, names of foodstuff and other tangible things

6. Ama—   **ama**khanda   (heads)

Other nouns in this class—amakhabe (watermelons), amaqolo (backs), amajazi (jackets); plural form of nouns in class

7. Isi—   **isi**guli   (a patient)

Other nouns in this class—isitsha (a dish), isibhamu (a gun), isilwane (an amimal); depict more things

8. Izi— **izi**guli (patients)

Other nouns in this class—izitsha (dishes), izibhamu (guns), izilwane (animals); plural form of nouns in class 7.

9. i(m, n)— **im**pendulo (an answer)

Other nouns in this class—inkanyezi (a star), inkomazi (a cow), impilo (a life)—tangible possessions and concepts

10. izi(m, n)— **izim**pendulo (answers)

Other nouns in this class—izinkanyezi (stars), izinkomazi (cows), izimpilo (lives); plural form of nouns in class 9

11. u— **u**godo (a piece of wood)

Other nouns in this class ufa (crack), ubambo (rib), udebe (lip)—

12. izi(m, n)— **izin**godo (pieces of wood)

Other nouns in this class—izimfa (cracks), izimbambo (ribs), izindebe (lips), plural forms in class 11.

14. Ubu— **ubu**so (a face)

15. Uku— **uku**dla (food)

16. uku— **uku**fa (death)

From the above classes of nouns

Translation of nouns in both singular and plural forms

Body parts

<u>Singular Form</u>   <u>Plural form</u>

Singular Form	Plural form
▪ Head	Heads
Ikhanda	Amakhanda
Inhloko	Izinhloko
▪ Neck	Necks
Intamo	Izintamo
Umqala	Imiqala
▪ Trunk/body	Trunks/bodies
Umzimba	Imizimba
▪ Arm or the whole upper limb	
Ingalo	Izingalo
▪ Hand	Hands
Isandla	Izandla
▪ Chest	Chests
Isifuba	Izifuba
▪ Abdomen or stomach	
Isisu	Izisu

- Whole lower limb

Umlenze   Imilenze

- Thigh   Thighs
Ithanga (ilithanga)   amathanga

- Leg (lower part of the lower limb) Legs
Umbala   Imibala
Isitho   Izitho

- Foot

Unyawo   Izinyawo

From above one can make a note that when words are changed to the plural form the prefix is the part of the word that goes through changes as opposed to English where an addition of suffix (-s or -es) is usually the case.

Taking a closer look at the words and how they transform between the two forms; note the following:

Nouns usually start with an i—or a u-. they actually start with an in-/is/ ili—or um-/ulu and its nor apparent for all of them.
To transform words to a plural in isiZulu means you leave the trunk of the word unchanged and alter the prefix. It happens as follows:

Singular Form   Plural form
In—   Izin-
Is-/isi   Iz-/izi
Ili—   Ama-

Umu—	Imi-
U-/Ulu—	Izi-/izin-/izim-
Umu—	Aba-
U—	O-

The shaded examples have not been illustrated here are some examples to illustrate; note the bold and underlined:

- Nail (fingernail)

Uzipho (**ulu**zipho)   **Izin**zipho

- Human being

Umuntu   **Aba**ntu

- Grandmother

Ugogo   **O**gogo

Working out plurals for words may be challenging but given time it becomes part of everyday use. Some generalizations can be made (1) objects normally start with i-/in-/ili or i—and they transform to izi-/izin—or ama respectively.

As expected some words do not conform to the above conversions (uncountable nouns), it is either they come in plural form or they start with ubu- or uku-.

Examples

Food—   Ukudla

Death—   Ukufa

Face (noun)—   Ubuso

Milk—   Ubisi
Humanity—   Ubuntu
Water—   Amanzi

(a plural exists for a drop and drops of water)
Iconsi lamanzi—amaconsi amanzi

Another point of note is that nouns **always** start with vowel in isiZulu, if one does not know the preceding vowel one cannot work out the plural form.

On the head

Singular Form   Plural form

- Face
Ubuso   —

- Forehead
Isiphongo   iziphongo

- One lock of hair and hair
Unwele   Izinwele

- Eye
Ihlo (ilihlo)   Amehlo

- Ear
Indlebe   Izindlebe

- Nose

Ikhala   amakhala

- Cheek

Isihlathi   Izihlathi

- Mouth

Umlomo   Imilomo

- Tooth

Izinyo   Amazinyo

- Lip

Udebe   Izindebe

Other organs and internal organs

Please note that the author worked out the names of internal organs from animal equivalents through the practice of slaughtering as internal organs of human are not explored otherwise. Their understanding is that of different types of meat.

Singular Form   Plural form

- Throat

Umphimbo   Imiphimbo

- Lung

Iphaphu   Amaphaphu

- Heart

Inhliziyo   Izinhliziyo

- Liver

Isibindi   Izibindi

- Intestine(s)

Ithumbu   Amathumbu

- Stomach (the actual organ)

Usu

- Pancrease

Impundu   Izimpundu

- Gall bladder

Isigubhu senyongo   Izigubhu zenyongo

- Spleen

Ubende   —

- Urinary bladder

Isigubhu somchamo   Izigubhu zomchamo

In essence the word bladder means container/bag which is "isigubhu" in isiZulu the other words describe the contents

Gall/bile—inyongo

Urine—Umchamo

PRONOUNS

POSSESSIVE PRONOUNS.
The following are possessive pronouns, their verb and adjective prefixes have also been included in the sentences that are used as examples.

Mina—me/I
I am wearing a blue shirt. e.g. Mina **ngi**fake iyembe elihlaza. (used with a verb)

Thina—us/we
e.g. Thina **si**hlezi emnyango. (used with a verb) We are seated near the door.

Wena—you (to one person)
e.g. **Wena** uhlangane nemibuzo enzima.(used with an adjective) You were faced with difficult questions.

Nina—you (to more than one person)
e.g. Nina **niba**ngaka kanti. (used withan adjactive)
In certain cases an agreeing prefix is ni—and the (ba) falls out as shown in the following example.

Nina **ni**njani? How are you?

Time and times
Long time—isikhathi eside
Many minutes—imizulu eminingi
Long hours—amahora amade

A lot of times/many occasions—Izikhathi eziningi/ amahlandla amaningi

Refering to people of different age groups

Child—Umntwana/ ingane

Male child—ingane yomfana
           —umntwana womfana

Female child—ingane yentombazane
              —umntwana wentombazane

Boy—umfana
Girl—intombazane

In the mating stage/ when refered to by their parents/ when referred to by the partner
Boy—insizwa
Girl—intombi

Man—indoda
OR
Male person—umuntu wesilisa

Woman—umfazi (a lot of women take offense to the use of this word)
OR
Female person—umuntu wesifazane

Example of application
Female ward—iwadi labesifazane.

Old lady—isalukazi
Old man—ikhehla/ ixhegu

VERBS IZENZO

VERBS TEND NOT to make much sense when they are not in a sentence. Like nouns the trunk or the stem of the verb does not go through a lot of transformation rather the prefix says a lot about its subject.

The use of verbs and the description of a few shall be demonstrated in the different tenses.

TENSES—INKATHI YESENZO

I N ISIZULU THE tense of a sentence of a statement is represented in the verb. The verb has a trunk (isiqu) or a major part that contains its meaning. In most cases the trunk of the verb is not altered as it goes through changes in tenses.

Three sentences shall be used in all tenses as examples and alterations that occur are noted.

The sentences are:
In English:

1. The nurse is injecting the patient.
2. Girls are injecting the patient.
3. The doctor is examining the injured people.

Then in isiZulu (direct translation)

1. Unesi ujova isiguli.
   Here the verb is:—jova
   It has two syllables:—jo—and—va.

2. Amantombazane ajova isiguli.

3. Udokotela uxilonga abantu abalimele.
   Here the verb is: xilonga
   It has three syllables:—xi-,—lo—and—nga.

The present Tense (Inkathi yamanje)

1. **U**nesi **u**jova isiguli.

Please note that the prefix put in on the verb aggrees with the subject.
For interest's sake let us say a few girls were injecting the patient, the sentence would then look like this:

2. **Ama**ntombazane **a**jova isiguli.
3. **U**dokotela **u**xilonga abantu abalimele.

The present perfect tense (Inkathi ephelele)

Here it is just the conversion of the last vowel of the verb to an—e. The change is precisely that for almost all occasions, as our sentences shall illustrate.

1. Unesi ujov**e** isiguli.
2. Amantombazane ajov**e** isiguli.
3. Udokotela uxilong**e** abantu abalimele.

In certain circumstances all the vowels in the verb are replaced with an e. e.g.

Umalume u**lala** esibhedlela.

Becomes

Umalume u**lele** esibhedlala.

Thankfully the latter circumstances are rare and this is not necessarily an area of confusion.

The past Tense (Inkathi edlule)

1. Unesi **wa**jova isiguli.

Please note that it is only the prefix to the verb that has changed to put he sentence in the past tense.

2. Amantombazane **a**jova isiguli.

Please note that in written form the past tense and the present tense look identical but please listen carefully to the spoken or pronounced form.

3. Udokotela waxilonga abalimele.

The recent past tense (Inkathi esanda kudlula)

The element added in this case is a separate word to indicate that the occurrence is recent in its nature. The element added is a word, uqeda/usanda.

Here are the examples.

1. Unesi uqeda kujova isiguli
OR
1. Unesi usanda kujova isiguli.

2. Amantombazane aqeda kujova isiguli.
OR
2. Amantombazane asanda kujova isiquli.

3. Udokotela uqeda kuxilonga abalimele.
OR
3. Udokotela usanda kuxilonga abalimele.

There is an element of overlap between this tense and the present perfect tense. Some people prefer that the present perfect tense be used instead of the recent past tense.

The future Tense

It is rather important to note that the future tense is also divided into the eventual future tense and the further future tense. The difference is that the eventual future tense is more promising to happen while the further future tense is less so.

The eventual future tense (Inkathi ezofika)

An element of the future tense is added in the verb; observe its place of insertion.

1. Unesi u**zo**jova isiguli.
2. Amantombazane a**zo**jova isiguli.
3. Udokotela u**zo**xilonga abalimele

As it appears, it is merely the present tense with an addition of the element to indicate the future tense.
The further future tense (Inkathi eyofika)

An element of the future tense is also inserted in the sentences; again notice its position of insertion

1. Unesi u**yo**jova isiguli.
2. Amantombazane a**yo**jova isiguli.
3. Udokotela u**yo**xilonga abalimele.

There exists other tenses e.g. immediate past tense, remote past tense, past continuous tenses etc. Further detail on these is entirely for descriptive purposes and thus has been omitted.

NEGATIVE FORMS

THE NEGATIVE FORM of a sentence is denoted on the verb. The tense dictates what changes and modifications the verb undergoes to have the sentence in a negative form. The changes are showed in bold in the following sentences.

The sentences in English are:
1. Jabulani is sleeping in the hospital.
2. Louise is injured on the ear.
3. Philani is pushing the bed.
4. Grandmother is paying the rent.

Positive form in a present tense
1. UJabulani ulele esibhedlela.
2. U-Louise ulimele endlebeni
3. UPhilani uphusha umbhede.
4. Ugogo ubhadala intela.

Negative form in a present tense (the same sentences have been used)

1. UJabulani **ka**lele esibhedlela.
   OR
1. UJabulani **aka**lele esibhedlela.
   OR
1. UJabulani akalalanga esibhedlela.

2. U-Louise **ka**limele endlebeni.
   OR
2. U-Louise **aka**limele endlebeni.
   OR
2. U-Louise **aka**limala**nga** endlebeni

3. UPhilani **ka**phush**i** umbhede.
   OR
3. UPhilani **aka**phush**i** umbhede.
   OR
4. UPhilani akaphushanga umbhede.
   OR
4. Ugogo **ka**bhadal**i** intela.
   OR
5. Ugogo **aka**bhadal**i** intela.
   OR
5. Ugogo **aka**bhadala**nga** intela.

Take note of the "i" that replaces the last vowel in examples 3 and 4.

Positive form in the past tense
   1. UJabulani walala esibhedlela.
   2. U-Louise walimala endlebeni.
   3. UPhilani waphusha umbhede.
   4. Ugogo wabhadala intela.

Negative forms in the past tense.

   1. UJabulani **ka**lala**nga** esibhedlela
      OR
   1. UJabulani **akazange alale** esibhedlela.

2. U-Louise **ka**limala**nga** endlebeni.
   OR
2. U-Louise **akazange alimale** endlebeni.

3. UPhilani **ka**phusha**nga** umbhede.
   OR
3. UPhilani **akazange aphushe** umbhede.

4. Ugogo **ka**bhadala**nga** intela.
   OR
5. Ugogo **akazange abhadale** intela.

PROCESSESS AND STATES

E XAMPLES ARE USED to describe these.

PROCESS	STATE
1. Umama uyalala	Umama ulele
Sleeping	Asleep
Mother is sleeping.	Mother is asleep.
2. Ingalo iyakhathala uma ngiyiphakamisa.	Ingalo ikhathele.
Tiring	Tired
Raising my arm is tiring.	My arm is tired.
3. Inxeba lidinga ukuthungwa.	Inxeba lithungiwe.
Suturing	Sutured
The wound needs suturing.	The wound is sutured.

ADJECTIVES

THERE ARE TWO groups of adjective in isiZulu

Type I: Generally concerned with describing appearance, quantity and size.

Type II: Used more in description of character, colours and other various qualities.

The manner in which they are used is having the stem of the adjective in agreement with the noun or the subject it is used to describe.

Type I

A wide range of adjective stems are given, translated and a few put into use in a sentence.

-hlanu—five
-bili—two
-ningi—many
-dala—old
—de—long
-sha—new
—ne—four

-khulu—big
e.g. **Um**bhede **om**khulu uyasinda.
The big bed is heavy

-ncane—small
e.g. **I**-BP cuff **e**ncane ilahlekile.
The small BP cuff is missing.

-fushane—short
e.g. **I**-plaster **im**fushane.
The plaster is short.

OR

e.g. **I**naliti **em**fushane ingcono.
The short needle is better.

-thathu—three
e.g. **Ama**doda **ama**thathu alimele engozini yebhasi.
Three men were injured in the bus accident.

Type II

-mnyama—black
-njani?—how?
-qotho—responsible
-manzi—wet
-mhlophe—white
-nje/-njalo—like/like that
-luhlaza—green/blue
njengotshani—like the grass (green)
njengesibhakabhaka—like the sky (blue)

In isiZulu the word for colorblue = hlaza is used for both green and blue, to make a distinction "hlanza njengesibhakabhaka" to say blue or "hlaza njengotshani to say green.

-buhlungu—hurtful/painful
-ngakanani?—how much?
-mpofu—fair (in color, typically used to refer to the complexion of a persons skin)

-buthakathaka—weak
e.g. **Imi**lenze yami **i**buthakathaka.
My legs are weak.

-lula—easy/light
e.g. **Ngi**yenze **ka**lula i-procedure.
I went through the procedure easily.

—ngcono—better
e.g. **Ku**ngcono ukulala embhedeni.
It is better to sleep on the bed.

-mnandi—gratifying (enjoyable)/delicious
e.g. **Ama**hewu **a**mnandi.
Amahewu are delicious.

-muncu—sour
e.g. Idokwe ledayabhethi **limuncu**.
The diabetic soft porridge is sour.

LOCATIVES/PREPOSITIONS

FIVE PREFIXES ARE used to denote positions and locations.

o-

e-

ku-

kwa-

ki-

These shall then be put into sentence.

The prefix e—is the most commonly used to denote places and body locations etc.

Ngilimele ekhanda.
I am injured on the head.

Umama ngimushiye ewadini.
I left mother in the ward.

Ngivakashele ekhaya ngamaholide.
I visited home during the holidays.

The prefix o—is used when the name of the place starts with a vowel or when the preposition would otherwise would not agree with the use of prefex e-

Iziguli oLundi zisheshe zilulame.

Patients at ULundi recover quickly.

Kuyabanda **o**lwandle lwaseKapa.
It is cold in the ocean in the Cape.

The prefix ku—is used when a person's name, an object or an actual site is
going to be in mention as a locative or a preposition.

Isipopolo sami si**ku**Shabalala.
My binoculars are with Shabalala.

Ngimazise ukuthi ame **ku**layini.
I told him to wait on the queue.

Incwadi uyibeke **ku**-shelf yakhe.
He put the book on his shelf.

The prefix kwa—means the place of/belonging to.

Ngivakashele **kwa**malume izolo.
I visited my uncle's place yesterday.

The prefix ki—means in/inside/within/with. It is used with pronouns in
most cases.

Ipeni lakho li**ki**mi(na).
Your pen is with me.

Imvelophu ngiyithumele **ki**ni(na).
I sent the invelope to your place.

PUTTING THIS MANUAL INTO USE

DIFFERENT SECTIONS ARE going to be introduced in English, scenarios are going to be made and a conversation in isiZulu is going to be carried out. The conversations are predominantly going to be between Dr. Carlton, Khekheleza (a 26 year old female patient who speaks isiZulu), a family member of Khekheleza (her father Khumbula) and other patients in the health care setting with Khekheleza. Other introductions shall be made should there be other characters to enter the conversations.

THE GREETINGS

FOR GREETINGS AT any time of day, to one person e.g. a patient in the consultation room, a nursing sister or colleague etc.

Dr. Carlton: Sawubona
Khekheleza: Yebo

INTRODUCING YOURSELF

I AM DR. CARLTON.

Dr. Carlton: Ngingu dokotela Carlton.
OR
My name is Dr. Carlton
Dr. Carlton: Igama lami udokotela Carlton.

When greeting many individuals e.g. a patient and a family member, a group of nursing sisters, patients on the waiting queue, a group of collegues

Dr. Carlton: Sanibona OR Sanibonani.
Khekheleza & partner: Yebo.

To complete the greetings, with one person then you go

Dr. Carlton: Unjani?
Khekheleza: Ngiyaphila

With many individuals

Dr. Carlton: Ninjani
Khekheleza & partner: Siyaphila

Literal meaning is I am well

Other responses

Ngikhona, by one person (literal meaning—I am here)

Sikhona, by many people

IMPORTANT FINDING TO MAKE

I F THE PATIENT speaks isiZulu or knows it.
You may ask what they speak?

Dr. Carlton: Ukhuluma ini? OR Ukhulumani?
Khekheleza: IsiZulu
Khekheleza: seSotho/ seVenda / sePedi / isiXhosa / isiSwati / isiNdebele

If the response to what do you speak is isiZulu, you can proceed without difficulty.
If the response is isiSwazi, isiXhosa or isiNdebele you can proceed with an expectation of minor difficulties along the way.
If the response is any other language ask if they know isiZulu. Depending on the answer, expect some difficulty along the way. This is determined by how much a patient knows.

OR if they speak isiZulu
Dr. Carlton: Uyasikhuluma isiZulu?
Dr. Carlton:: Uyasazi isiZulu?

Other possible responses:

Khekheleza: Yebo
OR
Khekheleza: (nodding) Uhh-eeh

WELCOMING THE PATIENT

H AVING GREETED AND introduced yourself to the patient it is important to welcome them.

- Ask them their names

Dr. Carlton: Ubani igama lakho?
Khekheleza: Ukhekheleza
                            OR
Dr. Carlton: Wena ungubani?
Khekheleza: NginguKhekheleza

- Ask them to sit down (they may sit and thank you or just sit)

Dr. Carlton: Ngicela uhlale phansi.

                   OR for the easier way
Dr. Carlton: (Ngiyakucela) Hlala phansi.

To instruct a person to sit down

Dr. Carlton: Hlala phansi.

There are two ways of giving instructions that are illustrated above, asking and giving a direct order. Asking makes it sound polite, however if you sound polite an order sounds as good

The History

1. PERSONAL DETAILS

- Name?

Dr. Carlton: Ubani igama lakho?

Khekheleza: Ukhekheleza

OR

Dr. Carlton: Wena ungubani?

Khekheleza: Ngingukhekheleza

- Surname?

Dr. Carlton: Ungowakwabani?

Khekheleza: NgingowakwaKhumalo

OR

Dr. Carlton: Ubani isibongo sakho?

Khekheleza: UKhumalo.

- You can be quick and ask for name and surname.

Dr. Carlton: Igama nesibongo

Khekheleza: Khekheleza Khumalo

- Age?—How old are you?

Dr. Carlton: Unangaki?

Khekheleza: Ngina—24.

OR

Dr. Carlton: Uneminyaka emingaki?

Khekheleza: Ngineminyaka engu-24

OR

The response may be just a number

Khekheleza: 24

- Date of birth?

Dr. Carlton: Wazalwa nini?

Khekheleza: Ngo-1984/ 1984

Sometimes you may be asking a patient for their age only to find that they respond by giving you their year of birth. This is common with the older people who do not work out their ages but just remember the year of birth.

In which case they would answer as depicted in the following example:

Dr. Carlton: Unangaki?

Khekheleza: Ngingoka—84.

They do this so that you can work out their age by yourself. So don't listen out for the number and take it as you hear it.

- Place of residence?

Dr. Carlton: Uhlala kuphi?

Khekheleza: Ngihlala e-Orlando.

OR

Dr. Carlton: Uvela kuphi?

Khekheleza: Ngivela e-Orlando.

- Marital Status?—ask if they are married?

Dr. Carlton: Ushadile?

Khekheleza: Yebo, ngishadile.

OR

Khekheleza: Cha, angikashadi

Khekheleza: Cha, angishadanga/ Angishadile

Other responses: divorced

Khekheleza: Ngidivosile

Khekheleza: Ngihlukanisile

- Civil Status? Do you work?

Dr. Carlton: Uyasebenza?)

Khekheleza: Yebo

or Qha/ Cha/uhh-uhh

OR

Do you go to school?

Dr. Carlton: Uyafunda?

Khekheleza: Yebo

or Qha/ Cha/uhh-uhh

Khekheleza: Ngifunda e-Gugulethu High School.

OR

Are you a pensioner?

Dr. Carlton: Uhola impesheni?

Khekheleza: Yebo

or Qha/ Cha/uhh-uhh

- Handedness—Which hand do you use to eat?

Dr. Carlton: Usebenzisa isandla sangakuphi uma udla?

Khekheleza: Right /left.

OR

Do you use your right hand?

Dr. Carlton: Usebenzisa isandla sokudla?

Khekheleza: Yebo

or Qha/ Cha/uhh-uhh

2. Presenting Complaints

The patient may be asked in different ways why they have presented to the health setting.

- How can we help you?

Dr. Carlton: Singakusiza kanjani?

- How can I help you?

Dr. Carlton: Ngingakusiza kanjani?

- What do you want from the doctor?

Dr. Carlton: Ufunani kudokotela?

- Why are you here?

Dr. Carlton: Kungani ulapha?

- What is troubling you?

Dr. Carlton: Uhlushwa yini?

Or

Dr. Carlton: Uphethwe yini?

- Why are you here?

Dr. Carlton: Yinindaba ulapha?

- What brings you here?

Dr. Carlton: Ulethwe yini lapha?

> If you have used this question the mode of transportation may be the response with this question

Headache.

Khekheleza: Kubuhlungu ikhanda

Khekheleza: Ngiphethwe ikhanda.

OR many reasons—vomiting, painful knees, fever and weakness

Khekheleza: Ngiyahlanza, kubuhlungu amadolo, nginemfiva futhi ngibuthakathaka.

- Onset—from when?

Dr. Carlton: Kuqale/Kusukela nini?

OR

Khekheleza: Izolo

When did it start?

Dr. Carlton: Kuqale nini?

Khekheleza: Kuqale izolo.

Khekheleza: Kuthangi.

Time frames

Yesterday—Izolo

The day before yesterday—Kuthangi

Tomorrow—Kusasa

Last week/previous week—Iviki eledlule

Last month/previous month—ngenyanga edlule

Last year—Ngonyaka odlule

Last of last week—Two weeks ago

Last of last month—two months ago

Last of last year—Two years ago

- Duration—For how long?

Dr. Carlton: Kuthatha isikhathi esingakanani?

Khekheleza: Amahora amabili

The above question is likely not to be understood and hence misinterpreted. The best way is to say exactly what it is that you are referring to (the complaint e.g. the headache) and ask how long it lasts.

- Associated Features—What else is troubling you?

Dr. Carlton: Ikuphi okunye okukuhluphayo?

Khekheleza: Kubuhlungu intamo.

OR

Where else is the pain?

Dr. Carlton: Kubuhlungu kuphi futhi?

Khekheleza: Kubuhlungu intamo.

The following questions pertain to the headache.

- Aggravating Factors—What makes the pain worse?

Dr. Carlton: Yini eyenza kube buhlungu kakhulu

Khekheleza: Umsindo omkhulu.

- Relieving Factors—What makes it better?

Dr. Carlton: Yini eyenza kube ngcono

OR

Dr. Carlton: Yine eyenza kube-bhetha?

Some of the patients may understand but the first one is better

Khekheleza: Ukulala phansi.

- Severity—How painful is it?

Is it the worst headache you have ever had?

Dr. Carlton: Liyaqala ukuba buhlungu kanje?

Khekheleza: Yebo

or Qha/ Cha/uhh-uhh

Or—Does it wake you from sleep?

Dr. Carlton: Liyakuvusa uma ulele?

Khekheleza: Yebo)

or Qha/ Cha/uhh-uhh

Enquiring about severity of the complaint is crucial; it may be the difference in making a correct diagnosis. Further illustrations on how to ask this question appropriately shall be revisited under the different sub-headings.

3. PAST MEDICAL HISTORY

- Admission History—Have you ever been admitted into a hospital?

Dr. Carlton: Wake walala esibhedlela?

Khekheleza: Yebo

or Qha/ Cha/uhh-uhh

If the answer to the above question is yes, then find out when and the reason for admission

Dr. Carlton: Bekunini futhi yini isizathu?

Khekheleza: Ngo-1994 ngaphuka umlenze.

- Surgical History—Have you ever had an operation?

Dr. Carlton: Wake wenza i-operation?

OR

Dr. Carlton: Wake wahlinzwa?

Khekheleza: Yebo

or Qha/ Cha/uhh-uhh

Time of the surgical operation

Dr. Carlton: Wahlinzwa nini.

Khekheleza: Ngo-2001 (year of the operation)

- Reason for the operation—Where on the body and why?

Dr. Carlton: Kuphi emzimbeni futhi bekuyini isizathu?

Khekheleza: On the left thigh for a fracture of the femur. Ethangeni lakwa-left elaliphukile.

- Current Medical Illnesses:

Dr. Carlton: Unayo i-asthma?

Khekheleza: Yebo
or Qha/ Cha/uhh-uhh

Chronic Illnesses

Diabetes?—I-diyabhethisi?
OR ushukela? OR sugar-diabetes?

High blood pressure?—I-hayi bhladi? OR high high? OR I-BP?

Rheumatic heart disease: Heart Diseases? Isifo senhliziyo?

Epilepsy?—I-epilepsy? OR Fainting disease?—Isifo sokuquleka?
Fitting disease—Ama-fits

I-HIV/Aids?—HIV or ingculaza?

The HIV/AIDS illness
HIV—Human Immunosuppressive Virus—igciwane lesandulelangculaza
AIDS—Acquired ImmunoDeficiency Syndrome—ingculaza
It has many names that have been ascribed to it due to its stigmatised nature.
These are informal for most part and they keep on evolving. An example
of a few are:
Intsholongwane (kagawulayo)
Amagama amathathu
Umashayabhuqe
Z3

There is a also considerable crossover with other closely associated
languages that tend to take place e.g. *isifo sikagawulayo* which is isiXhosa

---

- Time of diagnosis—When did you find out about asthma?

Dr. Carlton: Bakwazisa nini nge-asthma?

Khekheleza: Eminyakeni emibili edlule.

Dr. Carlton: Wake waba ne-TB?

Khekheleza: Yebo

or Qha/ Cha/uhh-uhh

- If yes, ask when

Dr. Carlton: Nini?

Khekheleza: Ngo 2001.

- Previous testing for HIV.

Dr. Carlton: Wake wahlola i-HIV?

Khekheleza: yebo

Dr. Carlton: Nini?

Khekheleza: Ngo-June

Result?

Dr. Carlton; Yathini imiphumela?/Athini ama-results?

Khekheleza: HIV positive/ HIV negative.

CD 4 count?

Dr. Carlton: Ithini i-CD 4 count? OR Athini amasosha Omzimba?

Khekheleza: Angiyazi

- Current Medications:

Dr. Carlton: Usebenzisa yiphi imithi? /Uthatha maphi amaphilisi?

Khekheleza: I-glucophage yediyabhethisi.

- Allergies?

Dr. Carlton: Unawo ama-aleji?

OR

Dr. Carlton: Ikhona imithi ekugulisayo?

Khekheleza: Yebo, ngine-aleji yemithi yesalfa

4. Family History

- Place of Birth—where were you born?

Dr. Carlton: Wazalelwa kuphi?

Khekheleza: E-Namibia e-Windhoek.

- Family structure:

Dr. Carlton: Ngicela ungazisa ngomndeni wakho.

Khekheleza: There is my mother, my brothers and sisters.—Kunomama nobhuti nosisi/ Kunomama nabafowethu nodadebethu.

- Parents:—Are your mother and father still alive? (if the question is appropriate)

Dr. Carlton: Ubaba nomama basaphila?

Khekheleza; Umama usaphila kodwa ubaba ushone ezinyangeni ezingu-6 ezedlule.

Dr. Carlton: Wadluliswa yini ubaba wakho?

Khekheleza: I-cancer yamaphaphu.

- Who do you stay with?

Dr. Carlton: Uhlala nobani?

Khekheleza: Nabantwana.

Relationships

Mother—Umama

Father—Ubaba

Child—Umntwana

Children—Abantwana

Uncle.—Umalume.

Aunt. = Umalumekazi (or u-anti)

Grandmother. = Ugogo (ukhulu—only used in certain areas)

Grandfather.—Umkhulu

Cousin.—Umzala

Nephew/niece. Umshana.

Grandchild.—Umzukulu.

Friend.—Umngani/ umkhozi

- Please tell me their names and ages.

Dr. Carlton: Ngicela ungazisa amagama neminyaka yabo.

Khekheleza: U-Brenda ona 12, no-Ringo ona 3

- Medical illness that they may be suffering from?

Dr. Carlton: Kukhona ukugula okubahluphayo?

Khekheleza: Yebo u-Brenda une-asthma.

- Family anomalies & disabilities:

Dr. Carlton: Ukhona okhubazekile ekhaya?

Khekheleza: Yebo, u-Robin wazala engenazo izinyawo.

- Hereditary illnesses in the family:

Dr. Carlton: Kukhona ukugula okuhambisana nabantu bomndeni wakho?

Khekheleza: Yebo, ubaba nomalume babengama-albino.

- How is your mother coping with your father's death?

Dr. Carlton: Kumphethe kanjani ukushona kukababa umama?

Khekheleza: Usengcono manje.

5. SOCIAL, OCCUPATIONAL HISTORIES AND HABITS.

- State of place of residence—How many rooms do you have in your house?

Dr. Carlton: Inama-rooms/ kamelo/gumbi amangaki indlu yakho?

Khekheleza: Angu-5 kanye nelokugezela.

- What is your house built of?

Dr. Carlton: Yakhiwe ngani indlu yakho?

Khekheleza: Yakhiwe ngotshani.

OR

Dr. Carlton: Uhlala endlini yothayela noma yesitina?

Khekheleza: Ngihlala endlini yesitina.

- Water and sanitation—Do you have taps in the house? [running water creates confusion]

Dr. Carlton: Zikhona izimpompi endlini?

Khekheleza: Cha/Qha

- How far do you travel to get water?

Dr. Carlton: Uhamba ibanga elingakanani ukuyokha amanzi?

Khekheleza: Amamitha angu-20.

> There is tendency to use equivalent distances as examples, e.g. from the door to the gate instead of distances in meters

- Where do you fetch water?

Dr. Carlton: Uwakha kuphi amanzi

Khekheleza: Ethangini lomphakathi.

- Environment and pollution:

Dr. Carlton: Uhlala edolobheni noma elokishini noma epulazini?

Khekheleza: Ngihlala ematshotshombeni.

- Soil or water pollutents in the area?

Dr. Carlton: Zikhona yini izinto ezidala ukungcola komoya, umhlabathi noma amanzi asendaweni?

Khekheleza: Yebo, kwakunemayini yamalahle eduze nendawo futhi udoti wayo usayingcolisa inhlabathi.

- Occupation: What do you do at work?

Dr. Carlton: Yini oyenzayo emsebenzini?

Khekheleza: Ngingumdayisi we-furniture.

Dr. Carlton: Unesikhathi esingakanani usebenza?

Khekheleza: Ngino-4 years.

- Habits—smoking?

Dr. Carlton: Uyabhema?

Khekheleza: Yebo

- When did you start smoking?

Dr. Carlton: Waqala nini ukubhema?

Khekheleza: Eminyakeni emibili edlule.

OR

Dr. Carlton: Kusukela nini?

Khekheleza: Ngo-2001

- How many cigarettes do you smome in a day?

Dr. Carlton: Ubhema osikilidi abangaki ngelanga

Khekheleza: Abahlanu/ 5 or five.

- Do you drink alcohol?

Dr. Carlton: Uyabuphuza utshwala?

Khekheleza: Yebo

- How many glasses do you drink in a week?

Dr. Carlton: Uphuza izingilazi ezingaki ngeviki?

Khekheleza: Amabhiya angu-5 nge wikhendi / ngempelasonto.

- What type of alcohol do you drink? (wine, beer, traditional beer, spirits etc.)

Dr. Carlton: Uphuza luphi uhlobo lotswala? (iwayini, ubhiya, utshwala besintu)

Khekheleza: Amabhiya.

- Do you use any other drugs?

Dr. Carlton: Uyazisebenzisa ezinye izidakamizwa?

Khekheleza: Yebo, i-zol uma ngibhema sometimes.

- Do you play any sport?

Dr. Carlton: Ukhona umdlalo owudlalayo?

Khekheleza: Yebo ngidlala i-ice hockey.

6. GENERAL HEALTH

- Appetite—Do you still like eating as much as you used to?

Dr. Carlton: Usakuthanda ukudla?

Khekheleza: Qha, sengidla ingxenye yokudla manje

OR

How much do you eat?

Dr. Carlton: Udla kangakanani?

Khekheleza: Ngidla kancane.

- Weight—weight loss?

Dr. Carlton: Unciphile emzimbeni?

Khekheleza: Yebo ibhulukwe lami liyangixega manje.

- Immunisations—Did you get immunised as a child?

Dr. Carlton: Wagoma ngenkathi usengumntwana?

Khekheleza: Angazi

- Travel history—When last did you go abroad?

Dr. Carlton: Ugcine nini ukuya phesheya?

Khekheleza: Ngangise-Mozambique ngo-Februwari.

- Impact of illness on patients' life

Dr. Carlton: Ukugula kukuthikameze kanjani?

Khekheleza: Kungihambise e-clinic, nomunye udokotela manje sengilapha.

Dr. Carlton: Kukhona okunye ofisa ukukhuluma ngakho noma ukubuza?
Khekheleza: Cha, kuphelele.

7. SYSTEMS REVIEW

I. CARDIOVASCULAR SYSTEM

- Have you had any pain or pressure on the chest?

Dr. Carlton: Uke waba nobuhlungu noma ukucindezeleka esifubeni.
Khekheleza: Cha

- Do you get short of breath on exertion?

Dr. Carlton: Uyaphelelwa umoya uma usebenza?
Khekheleza: Yebo, uma kubhokile ukukhwehlela.

- Have you ever woken up at night short of breath?

Dr. Carlton: Wake wavuka ubusuku uzizwa uphelelwa umoya?
Khekheleza: Yebo, nginokuvuka ngicinene.

- Do you get short of breath when lying flat?

Dr. Carlton: Uyakuphelela umoya uma ulala phansi?
Khekheleza: Yebo, sengize ngilala ngomqamelo omkhulu.

- How many pillows do you use when you sleep?

Dr. Carlton: Usebenzisa imiqamelo emingaki uma ulala?
Khekheleza: Emibili

- Are your ankles swollen?

Dr. Carlton: Zivuvukile izinyawo?

Khekheleza: Zinokuvuvuka uma ngime isikhathi eside.

- Do you have pain on your legs when you exercise?

Dr. Carlton: Bukhona ubuhlungu ezinyaweni uma uzivocavoca?

Khekheleza: Yebo uma ngicaca izitebhisi.

- Do you have cold blue hands/ feet?

Dr. Carlton: Ingabe izandla noma izinyawo zakho ziyabanda futhi ziluhlaza?

Khekheleza: Cha.

II. RESPIRATORY SYSTEM

- Are you ever short of breath?

Dr. Carlton: Uphelelwa umoya?

Khekheleza: Yebo ngizizwa ngivalekile

- Do you have a cough?

Dr. Carlton: Uyakhwehlela?

Khekheleza: Yebo

- Do you cough up anything?

Dr. Carlton: Kukhona okuphumayo uma ukhwehlela?

Khekheleza: Yebo, isikhwehlela esimhlophe.

- Do you cough up blood?

Dr. Carlton: Liyaphuma igazi uma ukhwehlela?

Khekheleza: Ngezinye izikhathi.

Colors

Please note that you can get away with using English names to talk about colors e.g.

white, black, yellow. red etc. Use common/ basic colors because some colors are easily mixed up. Beware that some people do not know about colors and rather use objects that may have a similar color to point at.

A few color translation are:

White—mhlophe

Black—mnyama

Red—bomvu/ bovu

Green—luhlaza okotshani

Blue—luhlaza okewsibhakabhaka

Yellow—phuzi

- Snoring?

Dr. Carlton: Uyahona?

Khekheleza: UBrenda uthi ngiyahona.

- Noisy breathing?

Dr. Carlton: Ukhona umsindo uma uphefumula?

Khekheleza: Cha

- Fever?

Dr. Carlton: Une-fever?

Khekheleza: Cha

Some patients may not know what fever is.

- Night sweats?

Dr. Carlton: Uyajuluka ebusuku?

Khekheleza: Yebo, ngize ngikhumule nezingubo.

- Previous pneumonia or TB?

Dr. Carlton: Wake waba ne-pneumonia noma i-TB?

Khekheleza: Yebo, i-TB.

> If the patient does not know what TB is use this:
> TB—chest disease—isifo sofuba

- When?

Dr. Carlton: Kwakunini?

Khekheleza: Ngo-2001

- Recent chest X-ray?

Dr. Carlton: Uke wathatha i-X-ray yesifuba muva-nje.

Khekheleza: Cha

III. GASTROINTESTINAL SYSTEM

- Heartburn?

Dr. Carlton: Unesilungilela?

Khekheleza: Uma ngidle kakhulu nangenkathi ngikhulelwe.

- Indigestion?

Dr. Carlton: Unaso isilungilela?

Khekheleza: Cha

- Difficulty swallowing?

Dr. Carlton: Unayo inkinga nokugwinya?

Khekheleza: Yebo, kubuhlungu.

- Solids or liquids.

Dr. Carlton: Uyakhona ukugwinya amanzi?

Khekheleza: Yebo, futhi akubuhlungu.

Dr. Carlton: Kuba buhlungu uma ugwinya inyama?

Khekheleza: Yebo, uma ngingayihlafunanga kahle.

- Nausea and or vomiting?

Dr. Carlton: Uke wazizwa kuthi hlanza noma uke wahlanza?

Khekheleza: Yebo, ngike ngizwe kuthi ngingahlanza.

- Vomited?

Dr. Carlton: Uke wahlanza

Khekheleza: Cha

- What do you vomit?

Dr. Carlton: Uhlanza ini?

- Have you vomited blood?

Dr. Carlton: Uke wahlanza igazi?

Khekheleza: Cha

- Bowel incontinence?

Dr. Carlton: Uyahluleka ukuzibamba noma ukuphunyuka?

Khekheleza: Cha

A BETTER QUESTION TO ASK IS . . .

Do you have accidents and mess yourself up?

Dr. Carlton: Uyaphunyuka uzimoshe?

Khekheleza: Cha

- Blood in your faeces?

Dr. Carlton: Uke waba negazi emasimbeni/ emakakeni?

Khekheleza: Khekheleza: Cha

- Abdominal pain?

Dr. Carlton: Unabo ubuhlungu besisu?

Khekheleza: Cha

- Altered bowel habits?

Dr. Carlton: Zishintshile izikhathi zakho zokuya endlini encane muva-nje?

Khekheleza: Cha

- Altered color of stool/faeces?

Dr. Carlton: Lukhona ushinto kumbala wamakaka akho?

Khekheleza: Cha

- Jaundice?

Dr. Carlton: Amehlo kanye nesikhumba sakho kwake kwaba phuzi?

Khekheleza: Yebo, ngonyaka odlule.

—Response: yes/no or a story
- Diet?

Dr. Carlton: Ngazise ngezidlo zakho zamuva-nje?

Khekheleza: Ngijwayele ukudla iphalishi nemifino.

- Peptic ulcerative diseases?

Dr. Carlton: Ayakuhlupha ama-ulcer esiswini?

Khekheleza: Cha

Other Gastrointestinal disease of note

The patients are usually aware of disease if they have had personal or close to personal contact with them.

Hepatitis—i-hepatitis

Colitis—i-colitis

Bowel cancer—i-cancer yamathumbu

OR

Cancer—umdlavuza

So for the above statement:

Bowel cancer—umdlavuza wamathumbu.

IV.   GENITOURINARY SYSTEM

URINARY

- Pain on passing urine?

Dr. Carlton: Uke waba nobuhlungu uma uchama?

Khekheleza: Yebo, ngizwa umchamo ungishisa.

- Getting up at night to pass urine?

Dr. Carlton: Uyavuka ebusuku uyochama?

Khekheleza: Yebo, kakhulukazi uma ngiphuze itiye ebusuku.

- Passing larger amounts of urine?

Dr. Carlton: Uchama umchamo omningi kunokujwayelekile? OR

Dr. Carlton: Uchama kakhulu?

Khekheleza: Cha

- Passing smaller amounts of urine?

Dr. Carlton: Uchama umchamo omncane kunokujwayelekile? OR

Dr. Carlton: Uchama imbijane?

Khekheleza: Cha

- Passing urine more frequently than usual?

Dr. Carlton: Uchama kaningi kunokujwayelekile?

Khekheleza: Cha

Quantities and Amounts

This basically relates to countable nouns (and objects) and uncountable nouns (and objects). These are intrinsically indistinct and tend to require a more in-depth understanding of language to master.

Augmentation/Increase

For countable objects e.g. vacoliters, jelcos, chairs, rooms etc. The relationship is as follows

A lot/Many—ningi

Big—Khulu

Put into context:

Many jelcos—ama-jelco amaningi

A big jelco—I-jelco enkulu.

For uncountable objects e.g. water, blood, pain etc. The relationship is as follows

Very intense (for pain)—kakhulu

A lot—ningi

Diminution/Decrease

For countable objects the relationship is as follows

A few—imbijane/ ezimbalwa

For uncountable objects

Not so intense (for pain)—kancane

Small size—ncane

The confusion merely stems from the fact that countable objects are not simply many in number but they can be big and uncountable objects are not simply big or small but can be subject to countable packaging or a quantifiable state. An example is that a lot of water does not just mean water in a big drum but can also mean water in many small glasses.

Other examples

Many small (sized) jelcos—ama-jelco amancane amaningi

A few big (sized) jelcos—amajelco amakhulu ayimbijane.

Bleeding a lot—Ukopha kakhulu.

Bleeding from many sites—Ukopha ezindaweni eziningi.

A lot of pain (intense pain)—Ubuhlungu obukhulu

Mild pain—Ubuhlungu obuncane.

Pain on a few sites—Ubuhlungu ezindaweni ezimbalwa/eziyimbijane

Pain at many sites—Ubuhlungu obuningi/ ubuhlungu ezindaweni eziningi.

- Urine colour change?

Dr. Carlton: Ushintshile umbala womchamo wakho?

Khekheleza: Yebo, usu-brown.

- Colour of urine?

Dr. Carlton: Unjani umbala womchamo wakho?

Khekheleza: Brown.

- Blood in your urine?

Dr. Carlton: Uke waba negazi emchanyeni?

Khekheleza: Cha

V.   VENEREAL

- Problems with sex life?

Dr. Carlton: Uke waba nezinkinga zocansi?

Khekheleza: Cha

- Rashes or lumps on genitals?

Dr. Carlton: Uke waxwaya ukuqubuka noma amaguludla ngasesithweni sangasese?

Khekheleza: Yebo, ngike ngaba ne-rash okuthiwa i-herpes.

- Sexually transmitted diseases?

Dr. Carlton: Wake waba nesifo esisithathelana ngokocansi?

OR

Dr. Carlton: Wake waba ne-STI?

Khekheleza: Yebo, bathi i-herpes i-STI.

As the enveloping work STI includes a number of diseases it may be more appropriate to break things down and ask more specifically about individual conditions.

Genital ulcers and genital growths

Do you have ulcers or abnormal growth on your sex organ?

Dr. Carlton: Kukhona izilonda noma okukhulayo okungajwayelekile isithweni socansi?

Khekheleza: Cha.

VI. Genital Discharge.

Do you have any fluid discharging from your sex organ?

Dr. Carlton: Kukhona okunguketshezi okuphuma esithweni socansi?

Khekheleza: Yebo

What color is it and how does it smell?

Dr. Carlton: Unjani umbala wako futhi kunuka kanjani?

Khekheleza: Ku-yellow, kunephunga elibi.

- Kidney stones?

Dr. Carlton: Wake waba namatshe ezinso/ kidney stones? OR

Dr. Carlton: Wake waba nama-kidney stones?

Khekheleza: Cha

MALE SPECIFIC

- Delay before passing urine?

Dr. Carlton: Kukuthatha isikhathi ukuthi uqale ukuchama?

Khumbula: Yebo, ngima isikhathi ngilinde umchamo.

- Dribbling in the end of urination?

Dr. Carlton: Ingabe kunokuconsa komchamo uma usuqedile ukuchama.

Khumbula: Yebo, ngizwa ngathi umchamo awukapheli.

- Difficulty in obtaining or maintaining an erection?

Dr. Carlton: Uke waba nenkinga yokuvukelwa noma ukulalelwa induku?

Khumbula: Yebo, induku yami ayisena-power.

FEMALE SPECIFIC

- Last normal menstrual period?

Dr. Carlton: Ugcine nini ukuya esikhathini? OR

Dr. Carlton: Ugcine nini ukuya emalangeni?

Khekheleza: Evikini eledlule.

- Age at first mentrual period?

Dr. Carlton: Wabe unangaki ngesikhathi uqala ukuya esikhathini?

Khekheleza: Thirteen

- Regularity of menstrual periods?

Dr. Carlton: Ingabe izikhathi zakho zokuya esikhathini zilandelana kahle?

Khekheleza: Yebo, ngiya esikhathini njalo ngenyanga.

- Pain during menstrual periods?

Dr. Carlton: Ingabe unobuhlungu obukhulu uma uya esikhathini?

Khekheleza: Sometimes

- Excessive bleeding during menstrual periods?

Dr. Carlton: Ingabe wopha ngokweqile uma uya esikhathini?

Khekheleza: Angazi

Ask how many pads are used per day during a menstrual period?

Dr. Carlton: Usebenzisa ama-pads amangaki ngosuku?

Khekheleza: Four

And if the pads get very wet
How wet do your pads get?

Dr. Carlton: Aba manzi kangakanani ama-pads akho?

Khekheleza: Kancane.

VII. HAEMATOLOGICAL

- Easy bruising?

Dr. Carlton: Uba nama-bruise kalula?

Khekheleza: Cha

- Fever or shivers and shakes?

Dr. Carlton: Unayo imfiva noma ukuqhaqhazela?

Khekheleza: Yebo, ikakhulukazi ebusuku.

- Difficulty stopping a small cut from bleeding?

Dr. Carlton: Ingabe wopha ngokweqile emihuzukwaneni emincane?

Khekheleza: Cha

- Lumps under your arms, groin or neck regions?

Dr. Carlton: Uke waxwaya izindlala/amaguludla emakhwapheni, entanyeni noma ngasesithweni sangasese?

Khekheleza: Yebo, ekhwapheni lakwa-left.

- Clots in your legs or lungs?

Dr. Carlton: Wake waba namahluli emithanjeni yegazi yezinyawo noma emaphashini?

Khekheleza: Cha, abakaze bangazise.

- Excessive bleeding of gums on teeth-brushing?

Dr. Carlton: Ingabe izinsini zakho zopha ngokweqile uma uxubha?

Khekheleza: Yebo, uma ngixubha isikhathi eside.

VIII. MUSCULOSKELETAL

- Joint pain?

Dr. Carlton: Unabo ubuhlungu bamalunga noma ama-joint?

Khumbula: Yebo, ngihlushwa ngamadolo.

[Joint—ilunga]

- Stiff joints?

Dr. Carlton: Ingabe ama-joint akho aqinile?

Khumbula: Amadolo, ayinkinga enkulu.

- Joint swelling?

Dr. Carlton: Kuyenzeka ama-joint akho avuvuke?

Khumbula: Uma ngime isikhathi eside

- Skin rashes?

Dr. Carlton: Uke waba nokuqubuka muva-nje?

Khumbula: Cha

- Back pain?

Dr. Carlton: Uke waba nobuhlungu beqolo?

Khumbula: Uyisho entsweni, ungathi ubukade wazi ukuthi liyankenketha.

- Neck pain?

Dr. Carlton: Uke waba nobuhlungu bentamo?

Khumbula: Cha

- Drying and or reddening of eyes?

Dr. Carlton: Amehlo akho ake oma noma aba bomvu?

Khumbula: Cha, leli lakwa-left aliboni kahle.

- Dry mouth or mouth ulcers?

Dr. Carlton: Wake waba namalonda noma ukoma komlomo?

Khumbula: Cha, umlomo woma uma ngonyiwe kuphela.

- Gout?

Dr. Carlton: Wake waba ne-gout?

Khumbula: Cha, kodwa kukhona u-nurse emtholampilo owathi ngine-arthritis.

- Rheumatoid arthritis?

Dr. Carlton: Wake waziswa ngokuthi une-athritis?

Khumbula: Angazi, ngazi nje i-arthritis njengoba bengikade sengishilo.

- Do your fingers ever become painful and become white and blue in the cold?

Dr. Carlton: Uma kubanda iminwe yakho kuyenzeka ibe buhlungu, ibe mhlophe noma ibe luhlaza?

Khumbula: Cha, akukaze kwenzeke lokho.

IX.   ENDOCRINE SYSTEM

- Swellings on your neck?

Dr. Carlton: Uke waxwaya ukukhukhumala/ukuvuvuka entanyeni?

Khekheleza: Cha

- Trembling of the hands?

Dr. Carlton: Kuyenzeka izandla zakho ziqhaqhazele?

Khekheleza: Cha, ngiqhaqhazela uma kubanda noma ngithuke kakhulu.

- Hot or cold weather preference?

Dr. Carlton: Uzwana nendawo eshisayo noma ebandayo?

Khekheleza: Ngizwana nendawo ekahle.

- Thyroid problem?

Dr. Carlton: Wake waba nenkinga ne-thyroid gland yakho?

Khekheleza: Yebo, ngenza i-operation ye-thyroind ngiseyingane.

Dr. Carlton: Kuphi?

Dr. Carlton: Kwakunini?

Khekheleza: Angazi

- Diabetes?

Have you ever been diagnosed with diabetis?

Dr. Carlton: Wake waziswa ngokuthi unoshukela/ idayabhethisi?

Khekheleza: Cha, abakaze bangitshele.

- Too much thirst?

Dr. Carlton: Uke waba nokonywa okungajwayelekile muva-nje?

Khekheleza: Uuh-eeh (shaking head in disagreement)

- Easy fatigability?

Dr. Carlton: Ingabe ungumuntu ohlushwa ukukhathala?

Khekheleza: Cha, angisheshi ukukhathala.

- Passing urine in large amounts?

Do you find that you pass large amounts of urine than usual?

Dr. Carlton: Ingabe uchama umchamo omningi kunokujwayele?

Khekheleza: Cha.

- Passing urine more frequently than usual.

Do you think you are passing urine more frequently than usual?

Dr. Carlton: Ingabe uchama izikhathi eziningi?

Khekheleza: Cha.

- Weight loss

Are you noticed that you are losing weight?

Dr. Carlton: Ingabe uyancipha emzimbeni?

Khekheleza: Cha

- Changes in appearance, hair, skin or voice?

Dr. Carlton: Uke waxwaya ukuthi kunoshintsho endleleni obukeka ngayo, izinwele, isikhumba noma izwi?

Khekheleza: Cha.

- Excessive sweating?

Dr. Carlton: Uke waxwaya ukuthi ujuluka ngokweqile?

Khekheleza: Cha, ngijuluka kahle-nje uma kushisa.

X.   NEUROLOGICAL SYSTEM

- Headaches?

Dr. Carlton: Liyakuphatha ikhanda?

Khekheleza: Linokungiphathe nje.

- Memory problems?

Dr. Carlton: Unazo izinkinga nokukhumbula izinto?

Khekheleza: Ngingumuntu okhohlwayo ngokwemvelo.

- Concentrating?

Dr. Carlton: Unayo inkinga nokulandelelisisa izinto?

Khekheleza: Hhayi

- Fainting episodes/ fits?

Dr. Carlton: Wake waquleka noma waba nama-fits?

Khekheleza: Yebo, ngangisasesikoleni.

Dr. Carlton: Kwakunini?

Khekheleza: Kudala

- Hearing problems?

Dr. Carlton: Unayo inkinga ngokuzwa ezindlebeni?

Khekheleza: Cha, ngizwa kahle.

- Visual problems?

Dr. Carlton: Unayo inkinga nokubona?

Khekheleza: Cha ngibona kahle.

OR

Ask about eye problems?

Dr. Carlton: Unayo inkinga yamehlo?

Khekheleza: Cha, anginankinga yamehlo.

- Dizziness?

Dr. Carlton: Ingabe uphethwe isiyezi?

Khekheleza: Asingiphethe njengamanje.

OR

Are you feeling dizzy?

Dr. Carlton: Uzizwa u-dizzy?

Khekheleza: Uuuh-uuh (shaking head in disagreement).

- Weakness, numbness or clumsiness in the arms or your legs?

Dr. Carlton: Uke waba buthakathaka, ukuba ndikindiki noma ubudedengu bezandla noma izinyawo?

Khekheleza: Unikina ikhanda (i.e. shakes head)

Pins and needles—Inkwantshu

[Literal meaning of pins and needles—omakhanjana nezinaliti]

- Previous stroke?

Dr. Carlton: Wake washaya i-stroke?

Khekheleza: Cha

A better question to ask is:

Dr. Carlton: Wake waba nesifo sohlangothi?

Khekheleza: Cha

An even better question to ask is about weakness on the one side of the body:

Have you ever had weakness on one side of the body?

Dr. Carlton: Wake waba-weak ohlangothini lomzimba?

Khekheleza: Cha

Dr. Carlton: Kwakunini?

- Head injury?

Dr. Carlton: Wake waba nengozi ekhanda?

Khekheleza: Yebo, ngake ngashaywa itshe ekhanda sidlala.

Dr. Carlton: Kwakunini?

Khekheleza: Kudala,

Dr. Carlton: Waquleka?

Khekheleza: Cha

- Sleeping difficulties?

Dr. Carlton: Unayo inkinga nokulala?

Khekheleza: Cha ngilala kahle.

XI. DERMATOLOGICAL SYSTEM

- Skin rashes?

Dr. Carlton: Uke waba nokuqubuka kwesikhumba?

Khekheleza: Yebo, ngihlushwa yi-acne

- Skin discolorations?

Dr. Carlton: Uke waba nokushintshelwa umbala wesikhumba?

Khekheleza: Ngigqwalile njengamanje, ngishiswa ilanga.

- Skin reactions?

Dr. Carlton: Ingabe kukhona okungahambiselani nesikhumba sakho?

Khekheleza: Yebo,

- What is it?

Dr. Carlton: Yini?

Khekheleza: Insipho yokuwasha.

A section of specific history taking for different systems has been included. Redundacy is inevitable, i.e. in the following section on particular history taking because taking history only varies with the questions of concern of the clinician. If a part of the history has been skipped the user is advised to refer to the section of general medical history taking.

OBSTETRICS HISTORY

I T IS WORTHWILE to mention that in all sub-disciplines of medicine it is crucial to ascertain the following:

- Name of patient
- Age of patient
- Consent for questioning

The last component is usually implied by the patient's presence in the consultation rooms but in case of adolescents it may be an actual tie—breaker and a step to creating a trusting bond.

To ask for permission to precede wth history taking ask . . . .

Will there be a problem if I ask you questions about why you are here?

Dr. Carlton: Kungaba nenkinga uma ngikubuza imibuzo ngento ekulethe lapha?

Khekheleza: Cha, singaqhubeka.

Presenting Complaint

- It is important to ask as open a question as possible in this part of the history and to ensure the complaint is understood as everything else follows on from here

A similar format as in the general medical history can be followed.

History of Presenting Complaint

- This will differ slightly depending on the presenting complaint (see below) but follows a well defined structure:

  o Onset (same as in the medical history)
  o Periodicity

When does it bother you?
Dr. Carlton: Kukuhlupha nini?
Khekheleza: kufika kubuye kwedlule.

How often does it occur?
Dr. Carlton: Kaningi kangakanani?

A better question to ask in this case in the number of episodes in one day or one hour as appropriate.

How many times do you get it in one day/ one hour?
Dr. Carlton: Kukubamba/kukuhlupha izihlandla ezingaki ngosuku/ ngehora?

  o Duration
How long does it last?

Dr. Carlton: Kukuhlupha isikhathi esingakanani?

Khekheleza: Mhlawumbe imizuzu engu-30.

     ○   Recurrence

How long after it subsides does it take to come back again?

Dr. Carlton: Kubuya ngemuva kwesikhathi esingakanani uma kusakuyekile?

Khekheleza: Uma sekuphele amahora amathathu.

Past Obstetric History
    ▪   Gravidity and Parity

Have you ever been pregnant?

Dr. Carlton: Wake wakhulelwa?

Khekheleza: Yebo.

How many times have you ever been pregnant?

Dr. Carlton: Wake wakhulelwa izikhathi (izihlandla) ezingaki?

Khekheleza: Kathathu

How many live children do you have?

Dr. Carlton: Unabantwana abangaki abaphilayo?

Khekheleza: Ababili, ngamphunyuka lona ophakathi.

If the woman is pregnant it is at this point that you ask for the antenatal card to gather further information. If the woman has not booked with an antenatal clinic and is pregnant you can advise them about booking.

May I see you antenatal card?

Dr. Carlton: Ngicela ukubona i-card lakho le-antenatal clinic?

Khekheleza: Ngiyilibale ekhaya; ngizoza nayo ngesikhathi esizayo.

I advise you to book at your nearest clinic. The booking should normally be done as soon as one knows that they are pregnant.

Dr. Carlton: Ngikululeka ukuthi uyobhukha e-clinic (emtholampilo) wakho oseduze. Umuntu kumele abhukhe ngokushesha lapho ethola ukuthi ukhulelwe.

- Dates of deliveries

Please tell me their birthdates?

Dr. Carlton: Ngicela ungazise izinsuku zabo zokuzalwa?

Start with the oldest and end with the youngest.

Dr. Carlton: Uqale ngomdala ugcine nomncane.

Khekheleza: Kukhona oka—2002 noka-2005

- Gender of babies

Tell me the gender of your children, starting with the first and so on.

Dr. Carlton: Ngazise ngobulili babantwana bakho, uqale ngomdala kanjalo kanjalo.

Khekheleza: Omdala intombazane bese lona owesibili abe ngumfana.

- Length of pregnancies

Was there a child who was born before time (before nince months)?

Dr. Carlton: Ukhona umntwana owamuthola ngaphambi kwesikhathi (izinyanga ezingu-9)?

Khekheleza: Umfana wami ngamuthola ezinyangeni ezingu-7.

- Induction of labor/ spontaneous

Did the delivery occur spontaneous or was it induced?

Dr. Carlton: Ukubeletha kwaziqalela noma kwaqaliswa?

OR

Did the labour pains start by themselves?

Dr. Carlton: Ingabe imihelo yaziqalela?

Khekheleza: Yebo, imihelo yaziqalela.

o Normal Delivery?

Was your child born normaly?

Dr. Carlton: Umntwana wamuthola ngokujwayelekile?

OR

Were your children born normaly?

Dr. Carlton: Abantwana wabathola ngokujwayelekile?

Khekheleza: Lona wesibili ngamthola nge-operation (caesarian section).

Was there use of forceps?

Khekheleza: Cha.

Was there use of the vacuum?

Was your child suctioned out with the vacuum cup?

Dr. Carlton: Ingabe umntwana wamubeletha ngokumuncwa ngenkomishi ye-vacuum?

Khekheleza: Cha

Was your child born by operation (caesar/caesarian/ c-section)?

Dr. Carlton: Umntwana wamuthola ngokuhlinzwa/ngomthungo/ nge-operation/ (caesar/caesarian/ c-section)?

Khekheleza: Yebo, lona wesibili.

What was the reason?

Dr. Carlton: Kwakuyini isizathu?

Khekheleza: Bathi umntwana ukhathele (Fetal distress)

○ Weight of babies

How much did your child weigh after birth?

Dr. Carlton: Wayenesisindo esingakanani umntwana mhla ezalwa?

OR

What was your baby on the scale?

Dr. Carlton: Sasithini isikali somntwana?

Khekheleza: Kwakungu-2000 grams lona wesibili.

○ Miscarriages, abortions, termination of pregnancies

Have you ever lost your pregnancy?

Dr. Carlton: Wake waphunyukelwa isisu?

OR

Have you ever had a miscarriage?

Dr. Carlton: Wake waba ne-miscarriage?

Khekheleza: Yebo, ngaphunyuka isisu ngaphambi kokukhulelwa ingane yesibili.

When and how far pregnant were you?

Dr. Carlton: Kwakunini futhi wawunesikhathi esingakanani ukhulelwe?

Khekheleza: Ngo-2004, saphunyuka nginezinyanga ezintathu.

Have you ever taken out a pregnancy?

Dr. Carlton: Wake wakhipha isisu?

Khekheleza: Cha.

Have you ever done an abortion?

Dr. Carlton: Wake wenza i-abortion?

Khekheleza: Cha.

When and how far pregnant were you? (as is appropriate)

Dr. Carlton: Kwakunini futhi wawunesikhathi esingakanani ukhulelwe?

   o Complications before, during and after delivery

Were there problems before birth of your child?

Dr. Carlton: Zaba khona izinkinga ngaphambi kokubelethwa umntwana?

Khekheleza: Ngaba ne-STI kanye ne-discharge ngaphambi kokuba ngithole umntwana wesibili.

Were there problems during the birth of your child?

Dr. Carlton: Zaba khona izinkinga ngesikhathi ubeletha?

Khekheleza: Amanzi ashesha ukunqamuka ngemva kwalokho bathi umntwana ukhathele.

Were there any problems after the birth of your child?

Dr. Carlton: Kwaba khona izinkinga usubelethile?

Khekheleza: Ngagula kakhulu bangitshela ukuthi ngine-sepsis.

Menstrual History

   ▪ 1st day of last menstrual period

What was the date on the first day when you were having your last period?

Dr. Carlton: Dr. Carlton: Dr. Carlton: Bekungu mhla kabani ngesikhathi usesikhathini okokugcina.

Khekheleza: Bezingu-3 kuMeyi.

   ▪ Regularity of normal cycle

Do your periods come every month?

Dr. Carlton: Uya zinyanga zonke esikhathini?

Khekheleza: Yebo.

Do they skip some months?

Dr. Carlton: Ingabe ziyeqeka izinye izinyanga?

Khekheleza: Cha

Do you take longer than a month to go on a period?

Dr. Carlton: Ingabe kuthatha isikhathi esevile enyangeni eyodwa ukuthi uye esikhathini?

Khekheleza: Yebo, ngezinye izikhathi.

How many days longer than a month?

Dr. Carlton: Amalanga amangaki ukudlula enyangeni?

Khekheleza: Kuyehluka.

Do you take less than a month before you go on a period?

Dr. Carlton: Ingabe kukuthatha isikhathi esingaphansi kwenyanga ukuthi uye esikhathini?

Khekheleza: Cha.

How many days is it? (as appropriate)
- Was this a planned pregnancy?

Did you plan to fall pregnant?

Dr. Carlton: Ukuhlelile ukuthi ukhulelwe?

Khekheleza: Yebo.

- Previous contraception

Do you do family planning?

Dr. Carlton: Uyawuhlela umndeni?

OR

Do you do pregnancy prevention?

Dr. Carlton: Uya-preventer?

Khekheleza: Ngangijova ngase ngayeka ngesikhathi sengifuna ukubamba.

- Any antenatal problems thus far?

Do you have any problems your pregnancy?

Dr. Carlton: Kukhona okukukhathazayo ngoba ukhulelwe?

Khekheleza: Cha, angikaboni lutho kepha angazi ukuthi ubuza ngani kahle kahle.

[These broadly are about haematuria, antepartum haemorrhage, abdominal pains, abdominal trauma, vaginal discharge etc.]

Past Medical History

A format similar to taking a medical past medical history should be followed

- Current or past illnesses
- Hospital admissions
- Past surgeries

Drug History

- Prescribed medications
- Non-prescribed medications/herbal remedies
- Recreational drugs

Family History

- Medical conditions
- Obstetric complications

Social History

- Occupation

Where to you work?
Dr. Carlton: Usebenza kuphi?
Khekheleza: Kwi-firm yezingubo.

What do you do at work?
Dr. Carlton: Wenzani emsebenzini?
Khekheleza: Ngiyahlala ngithunge izingubo.

- Support network

Are you still together with the father of the child?
Dr. Carlton: Nisahlalisana nobaba womntwana?
Khekheleza: Yebo.

Are there other people who are going to help with taking care of the baby?
Like family?
Dr. Carlton: Bakhona abozokusiza ngokunakekela umntwana? Njengomndeni?
Khekheleza: Yebo bakhona, umama kanye nodadebethu.

- Smoking
- Alcohol

GYNAECOLOGAL HISTORY

Introduction

- Name of patient
- Age of patient
- Consent for questioning

Consent for questioning is implied; patients present to the doctor and expect some information to be acquired from them to aid with the treatment to their ailments.

Presenting Complaint

It is important to ask as open a question as possible in this part of the history and to ensure the complaint is understood as everything else follows on from here.

History of Presenting Complaint

This will differ slightly depending on the presenting complaint but follows an orchestrated structure:

- If pain is involved ascertain site, radiation (if any) and character etc.

Where is the pain?

Dr. Carlton: Kubuhlungu kuphi?

Khekheleza: La (pointing) ngasenzansi kwenkaba.

- Onset

When did it start?

Dr. Carlton: Kuqale nini?

Khekheleza: Kunamaviki amabili.

- Periodicity

Is it always aching or does it come and go?

Dr. Carlton: Kuhlala kubuhlungo noma kukubamba kubuye kukuyeke?

Khekheleza: Kuhamba kubuye nyanga zonke?

- Duration

How long does it last?

Dr. Carlton: kuhlala isikhathin esingakanani?

Khekheleza: Isinsuku ezine.

- Recurrence? (the difference between this and periodicity is essential to draw out)

Does it come back when efforts at relief have been made?

Dr. Carlton: Kubuya kubuye yini uma uzame ukukudambisa?

Khekheleza: Yebo, kuhamba isikhashana uma ngithathe amaphilisi ezinhlungu.

Menstrual History

- Menarche and menopause

How old were you when you had your first period?

Dr. Carlton: Wawuneminyaka emingaki mhla uya esikhathini okokuqala?

Khekheleza: Ngangina-15.

- 1st day of last menstrual period

What was the date when you had your first bleed on the last period?

Dr. Carlton: Bekungu mhla kabani ngesikhathi wopha okokuqala mhla usesikhathi okokugcina?

Khekheleza: 26 Septhemba.

OR

When was your last period?

Dr. Carlton: Bekuyizingaki mhla uya esikhathini okokugcina?

Khekheleza: Bephakathi komhla ka-26 no-29 Septhemba.

- Length of bleeding (days)

How many days do you normally bleed?

Dr. Carlton: Wopha izinsuku ezingaki ngokujwayelekile?

Khekheleza: Izinsuku ezine.

- Frequency

How long do you have in between periods?

Dr. Carlton: Kudlula isikhathi esingakanini ukuthi ubuyele esikhathini?

Khekheleza: Inyanga eyodwa.

- Regularity

Do you always have periods every month without disruptions?

Dr. Carlton: Uhlale uya esikhathini nyanga zonke ngaphandle kokuphazamiseka?

Khekheleza: Yebo, angeqisi.

- Bleeding between periods

Does it happen that you bleed when you are not having a period?

Dr. Carlton: Kuyenzeka wophe ungekho esikhathini?

Khekheleza: Cha.

- Bleeding after intercourse

Does it happen that you bleed after having sexual intercourse?

Dr. Carlton: Kuyenzeka ukuthi wophe uma uqeda ukuhlanganyela ocansini?

Khekheleza: Yebo.

- Nature of periods
  - Heavy?

The number of pads/tampons (tampons not so much a goood meausure) used in one day and the amount of liquid contained in them dictate the weight of the periods.

How many times do you change tampons on average when you are having a period?

Dr. Carlton: Uwashintsha kangaki ngelanga ama-pads uma usesikhathini ngokujwayelekile?

Khekheleza: Ngiwashintsha ka-4.

How wet (soiled) are your paids on average when you change them?

Dr. Carlton: Asuku emanzi kangakanani ama-pads uma uwashintsha?

Khekheleza: Asuke engemanzi kakhulu

The use of drawings can come in handy to work the previous question more precisely

Through attentiveness the author has discovered and would like to relay that the luxury of pads should not be generalised as some women still resort to using a piece of cloth (usually a towel-like in nature) to prevent menstrual blood from flowing.

- o Clots?

Do you ever have clots in you menses?

Dr. Carlton: Kuyenzeka kube namahluli uma usesikhathini?

Khekheleza: Yebo, ikakhulukazi emalangeni okuqala.

- o Flooding?

Does it happen that your menses flow excessively?

Dr. Carlton: Kuyenzeka ukuthi wophe ngokweqile uma esesikhathini?

Khekheleza: Yebo, kodwa akusizo zonke izikhathi.

Past Gynaecological History

- Gynaecological symptoms
- Gynaecological diagnoses
- Gynaecological surgery
- Abnormal smears

Past Obstetric History

These can be cited from the obstetric history section.

- Gravidity and Parity
  - Dates of deliveries
  - Length of pregnancies
  - Induction of labor/Spontaneous
  - Normal Delivery?
  - Weight of babies
  - Gender of babies
  - Complications before, during and after delivery

Past Medical History

- Current or past illnesses
- Hospital admissions
- Past surgeries

Drug History

- Prescribed medications
- Non-prescribed medications/herbal remedies
- Recreational drugs

Family History

In the following the ones not expanded on are dealt with in detail in the obstetric history section or the general history section.

- Medical conditions
- Gynecological conditions
- Malignancies

Has anyone in your family (aunts/mother's and father's side) had a cancer of the ovaries (uterus/cervix/breasts).

Dr. Carlton: Ukhona emndenini (omalumekazi, o-anti ngakumama noma ngakubaba) owake waba nomdlabuza wamaqanda (isinye/ umlomo wesinye/ amabele)

Khekheleza: Cha, angikaze ngizwe.

- consanguinity

Has there been an instance in your where a close family member married another?

Dr. Carlton: Kuke kwenzeka emndenini ukuthi abantu bashadane emndenini?

Khekheleza: Hhayi akukaze kwenzeke.

Social History

- Occupation
- Support network
- Smoking
- Alcohol
- Marital status
- Ranking

ANAESTHETIC HISTORY

The gathering of information for ascertaining anaesthetic risks is similar to gathering medical history.

Other important issues are:

1.) Ensuring that the patient understands the process of anaesthetics and the surgery.

This is done by explaining these to the patient and then asking them to explain it back to you.

Alternatively these processes could be explained to the patient on their own language if this is possible.

This is important to facilitate co-operation between the patients and the practitioners in the operating theatres.

2) Cardiovascular risk
3) Respiratory risk
4) Full stomach or other gastro-intestinal risk

When was the last time you had something to eat/ drink?
Dr. Carlton: Ugcine nini ukudla noma ukuthola okokuphuza?
Khekheleza: Ekuseni

What was the time?
Dr. Carlton: Bekungubani isikhathi?
Khekheleza: Ngo-9.

What did you eat and drink?
Dr. Carlton: Udle wase waphuza ini?
Khekheleza: Ngidle ama-sandwich ngase ngiphuza itiye.

How much did you eat/ drink?

Dr. Carlton: Udle/uphuze kangakanani

Khekheleza: Ngidle ama-sandwich amabili ngaphuza inkomishi eyodwa yetiye.

5) Drug history
6) Previous anaesthetic and surgical history

EAR, NOSE AND THROAT

The following subjects should be covered:

- Allergies/atopic disease

Do you have asthma?

Dr. Carlton: Unayo i-asthma?

Khekheleza: Angazi

Do you have allertgic rhinitis?

Dr. Carlton: Unayo i-allergic rhinitis?

Khekheleza: Angazi

Better questions to ask about allergic conditions is to ask if the patient experiences times of nose blocking during spring and summer or if they play with pets and if they get abnormal itchiness if they have been playing in the grass or the carpet and etc.

Do you get a stuffy/blocked nose during spring or summer?

Dr. Carlton: Kuyenzeka uhlushwe ukucinana uma kusentwasahlobo noma ehlobo?

Khekheleza: Yebo, ikakhulukazi entwasahlobo.

Do you have excessive itchiness if you have been playing on the grass or the carpet or if you have been playing with pets (cat or dog)?

Dr. Carlton: Kuba khona ukulunywa okweqile uma ubukade udlala otshanini noma ku-carpet noma uma ubukade udlala nesilwane sokufuywa (inja noma ikati)?

Khekheleza: Yebo, akusamele ngidlale otshanini.

- Smoking

Do you smoke?

Dr. Carlton: Uyabhema?

Khekheleza: Cha

- Is there someone who smokes at home?

Dr. Carlton: Kukhona obhemayo ekhaya?

Khekheleza: Yebo, umfowethu uyabhema.

- Is there someone who smokes at school/work?

Dr. Carlton: Kukhona obhemayo esikoleni/emsebenzini?

Khekheleza: Yebo, abantu bayazibhemela.

- Pets at home

Do you have pets at home?

Dr. Carlton: Ninazo izilwane zokufuywa ekhaya?

Khekheleza: Yebo zikhona.

- Do you have a cat at home?

Dr. Carlton: Ninalo ikati ekhaya?

Khekheleza: Cha, alikho ikati.

- Do you have a dog at home?

Dr. Carlton: Ninayo inja ekhaya?

Khekheleza: Yebo ikhona.

- Do you play with the dog?

Dr. Carlton: Uyadlala nenja?

Khekheleza: Cha, ihlala phandle futhi angidlali nayo.

- Occupation

—Where do you work?

Dr. Carlton: Usebenza kuphi?

Khekheleza: Emafemini ezingubo.

—What do you do at work?

Dr. Carlton: Wenzani emsebenzini?

Khekheleza: Ngiyahlala ngithunge izingubo.

—How long have you worked there?

Dr. Carlton: Ususebenze isikhathi esingakanani?

Khekheleza: Iminyaka emithathu.

—How does your illness (symptoms) differ in work and at home?

Dr. Carlton: Ukugula kwakho kuhluka kanjani uma usekhaya noma usemsebenzini?

Khekheleza: Kuyafana nje.

—Do you feel better when you are at your place of work?

Dr. Carlton: Uzizwa ungcono uma usemsebenzini?

Khekheleza: Kungconywana uma ngisekhaya.

—Do you feel worse when you are at your place of work?

Dr. Carlton: Uzizwa kukubi kakhulu uma usemsebenzini?

Khekheleza: Yebo, kodwa kancane.

- History of previous surgery
- Previous trauma
- General medical history
- Seasonal or daily variation in symptoms

How does your illness differ along the course of the day?

Dr. Carlton: Kuguquka kanjani ukuphatheka kwakho ngokuqhubeka kosuku?

Khekheleza: Kungcono ekuseni bese kubheda ntambama.

How does your illness differ along the course of the year?

Dr. Carlton: Kuguquka kanjani ukuphatheka kwakho ngokuqhubeka konyaka?

Khekheleza: Kuba kubi kakhulu entwasahlobo (ngoSepthemba nango-Okthoba).

PSYCHIATRIC HISTORY

The essential difficulty posed by psychiatric illness is the possibility of underlying thought and thought form disorder that shall lead to confusion in a person with minimal mastery of the language of the patient.

However a translated Folstein's mini-mental status examination has been provided. Caution should be exercised with this instrument in the illeterate as well as in a mentally compromised person.

The Mini-Mental Status Examination

Patient: Examiner:

Date: Score:

Component	Questions	Normal	Patient
Orientation			
To time . . .	What is the year? Imuphu unyaka esikuwo? OR Unyaka? OR be more hinting Ngu-two-thousand and bani manje?	1	
	What is the season? Yisiphi isikhathi sonyaka manje? Kusebusika noma kusehlobo manje?	1	
	What is the month? Iyiphi inyanga esikuyo? Inyanga?	1	
	What is the day? Usuku? OR Ulwesingaki?	1	

	What is the date? Ithini i-date/zingaki namhlanje?	1	
To place . . .	What country are we in? Iliphi izwe esikulo? Caution: the usual answer offered is the region of the country.	1	
	What province? Iyiphi e-phrovinsi? Iphrovinsi?	1	
	What town or city Iliphi idolobha? Idolobha?	1	
	What hospital? Igama lesibhedlela?	1	
	Which ward? Iliphi iwadi? Iwadi?	1	
Memory Registration			
	This is a pen, watch, table, paper, book, door, cupboard, shirt, window, etc (any three objects to have the patient rehearse) What are the objects that I have pointed out to? Leli ipeni, itafula, iphepha, ibhuku, isicabha (unyango), iyembe, iwindi Iziphi izinto esengizibalile?	3	

Attention and Calculation	Either serial of sevens: (this presents particular difficulty with the illiterate) A hundred minus seven (serially) for about five times. Noting whether the answers offered are correct or not. Ikhulu ngisusa okuyisikhombisa? NOMA Handrethi ngisusa seveni? OR Spelling: Spell the word "world" backwards. Pela igama elithi "world" uqale ekugcineni ugcine ekuqaleni?	5	
Memory-Recall			
	What are the names of the three objects we talked about? Uyazikhumbula izinto ebesizibala?	3	
Language			
	Point to two different objects (preferably different to the ones for memory registration and recall) What is this? And this? Yini le? Lena? Lokhu?	2	

Repeating a statement			
	Say after me: No ifs, ands or buts. Isho kanje: NO IFS, ANDS OR BUTS.	1	
Three-stage Command			
	Take this paper into your hand, fold it in half and put it on the floor. Thatha le phepha uligobe liphindeke kabili bese ulibeka phansi.	3	
Read and obey instructions			
	Offer a paper written "close your eyes" see if they obey the instruction. Funda bese wenza okubhaliwe: A paper written "VALA AMEHLO" The patient is expected to close their eyes	1	
Writing a sentence			
	Write a sentence, saying anything that you like on this paper, (offer paper and pencil/pen) Or alternatively have them write on here Sentence: Here is a pen and paper (offer as appropriate and deemed safe), write in any sentence of your choice. Nali ipeni nephepha bhala umusho osho into oyithandayo.	1	

Copy design			
	(the same piece of paper used to write in a sentence can be used to carry out the following task) Please copy the following design: OR Dweba umdwebo ofana nalo: 	1	

TAKING A COLLATERAL HISTORY

In this section the taking of a collateral history shall also be visited.

There are two approaches to taking a collateral history.

1. The complicated way—asking the collateral direct questions and informs them to answer on behalf of the patient of concern.
2. The easy way—referring to the patient as a third person

PAEDIATRIC HISTORY TAKING

In paediatrics the history taken is almost always collateral from the parents.

In the following scenario Khekheleza has presented with her month old son.

Find out the nature of the relationship

What is your name?
Dr. Carlton: Ubani igama lakho.
Khekheleza: UKhekheleza Khumalo.

How are you related (to him or her?)
Dr. Carlton: Uhlobene kanjani naye.
Khekheleza: Ngingumama wakhe.

Do you live together?
Dr. Carlton: Nihlala ndawonye?
Khekheleza: Cha, uhlala nogogo wakhe.

Name of the mother?

Dr. Carlton: Ubani igama likamama wakhe?

Khekheleza: Yimi.

Name of the father?

Dr. Carlton: Ubani igama likababa wakhe.

Khekheleza: UMdumiseni Nzinisa.

You may ask the reason why the mother is not there if the informant is not the mother.

(in this example the mother of the child is the one who brought the baby in for the consultation)

In a case where Khekheleza's child was brought in by her aunt Ntombezinhle the doctor would ask about the mother.

Where is the mother of the child?

Dr. Carlton: Ukuphi umama wontwana?

Ntombezinhle: UseGoli.

OR

Why is the mother of the child not here with the child?

Dr. Carlton: Kungani umama wontwana engekho lapha nomntwana?

Ntombezinhle: Usebenzela ngaseGoli.

How old is he or she (the child)?

Dr. Carlton: Unangakanani?

Khekheleza: Unenyanga eyodwa nezinsuku ezimbili.

OR

How many moths does he or she have?

Dr. Carlton: Unezinyanga ezingaki?

Khekheleza: Unenyanga eyodwa nezinsuku ezimbili.

OR if the child looks older

How many years and months does he or she have?

Dr. Carlton: Uneminyaka nezinyanga ezingaki?

Khekheleza: Unenyanga eyodwa nezinsuku ezimbili.

In isiZulu when talking about the third person it does not become apparent that they are either male or female as they are just referred to as them, so finding out the sex of the person or the child can be delayed until later say for example examination.

The history from here onwards carries on as a medical history with a few additions that pertain to paediatrics. The components of the history and their succession are a personal preference; an inclusion of all important components has been attempted.

Major complaint

What bring you here today?

Dr. Carlton: Nilethwa yini lapha namhlanje.

Khekheleza: Akadli kahle, uyakhathala ajuluke uma edla aphinde ashintshe abe hlaza ebusweni.

History of major complaint

Onset

When did it start?

Dr. Carlton: Uqale nini.

Khekheleza: Selokhu samphuma esibhedlela, kepha manje sekwenzeka sonke isikhathi uma edla.

Duration

For how long does it carry on when it is happening?

Dr. Carlton: Kuthatha isikhathi esingakanani uma kumuhaqile.

Khekheleza: Kuyadlula isigamu sehora.

Aggravating factors
What makes it worse?

Dr. Carlton: Kuqalwa yini.

Khekheleza: Kumqala uma edla noma ephuza, kubuye kwenzeke noma eleli ngesisu.

Relieving factors
What makes it better?

Dr. Carlton: Yini eyenza kube ngcono?

Khekheleza: Ukuba simyekise ukudla.

Severity
Though this is hinted by the fact that the mother decided to bring the child to hospital/to see a doctor, it may give an indication of a pattern if it is an ongoing problem.

Dr. Carlton: Kubi kangakanani

Khekheleza: Ngoba sekumenza nsuku zonke sekungikhathaza impela.

Systematic history
The location of the systems review is truly a matter of technique, others prefer to get the whole picture of the patient before exploring other issues in the background while a counter-argument by those who put it towards the end is that it fits in missing gaps and one really is not to fish by flooding a patient with irrelevant questions to begin with.

Skin

Does he/she have a problem of rashes?

Dr. Carlton: Unayo inkinga yesikhumba nama-rash?

Khekheleza: Yebo, anokuvela abuye aziphelele.

Eyes

Has he/she ever had an eye problem/infection?

Dr. Carlton: Wake waba nenkinga yamehlo noma i—infekshini?

Khekheleza: Cha angikhumbuli

The word infection may not be understood, asking about a discharging eye or a red eye may increase the yield.

Has he/she ever had a red or discharging eye?

Dr. Carlton: Wake waba nehlo elibomvu noma eliphuma ubovu?

Khekheleza Cha, akakaze.

Has he/she ever had a foreign body in the eyes?

Dr. Carlton: Wake wangenwa into ehlweni?

Khekheleza: Yebo, unokungenwa izilwane ezincane bese ngiziphephetha.

Ears, Nose and Throat

Does he/she get frequent colds?

Dr. Carlton: Ingabe ungumuntu ohlushwa umkhuhlane?

Khekheleza: Yebo, njalo nje unokukhwehlela.

Does he/she have a stuffy nose/ nose blocking?

Dr. Carlton: Unako ukucinana noma ukuvaleka amakhala?

Khekheleza: Yebo, ngimuzwe ephefumula kanzima.

Does he/she breathe using the mouth?

Dr. Carlton: Ingabe uphefumula ngomlomo?

Khekheleza: Yebo, uhlala ekhamisile muva nje.

Does he/she snore?

Dr. Carlton: Uyahona?

Khekheleza: Cha, kodwa emini uyazwakala uma ephefumula.

Does he/she have period of not breathing and then starts breathing again when asleep?

Dr. Carlton: Kuyenzeka yini ukuthi uma elele ame ukuphefumula?

Khekheleza: Bengingakakuqapheli/ bengingakakuxwayi.

Does he/she have a problem with hearing?

Dr. Carlton: Unayo inkinga nokuzwa?

Khekheleza: Angazi, kepha ngicabanga ukuthi yena uyezwa.

Teeth

When did he/she start erupting teeth?

Dr. Carlton: Uqale nini ukumilisa amazinyo?

Khekheleza: Ngeviki eledlule.

OR

How many months old was he/she when they started erupting teeth.

Dr. Carlton: Wayenezinyanga ezingaki mhla eqala ukumilisa amazinyo.

Khekheleza: Eziyisihlanu.

Was it the same time with other children his/her age?

Dr. Carlton: Kwakuyisikhathi esifanayo nezinye izingane ezilingana naye?

Khekheleza: Yebo.

Cardiorespiratory

Shortness of breath

Does he/she breathe heavily like one would breathe when out of breath?

Dr. Carlton: Ingabe uphefululela phezulu njengomuntu ophelelwa umoya?

Khekheleza: Yebo, unephika.

Chest pain

The following question is for older children who can speak.

Does he/she ever complain of chest pain?

Dr. Carlton: Kuyenzeka akhale ngobuhlungu esifubeni

Khekheleza: Yebo.

Wheezing

Does he/she have noisy breathing?

Dr. Carlton: Kunomsindo yini ukuphefumula kwakhe?

Khekheleza: Yebo, uyanswininiza.

Syncope

Has the child (he/she) ever fainted?

Dr. Carlton: Wake waquleka umntwana?

Khekheleza: Cha.

Did he/she have jerky movements when they fainted?

Dr. Carlton: Ingabe wadlikiza/wadikiza mhla equleka? (showing fitting motions)

Khekheleza: Cha, ingalo yakwa-right yodwa eyayinyakaza.

For how long did he/she stay asleep when they collapsed?

Dr. Carlton: Walala isikhathi esingakanani elele mhla equlekile?

Khekheleza: Imizuzu emithathu kuya kwemihlanu.

Gastrointestinal

Vomiting

Is he/she vomiting?

Dr. Carlton: Uyahlanza/uyabuyisa?

Khekheleza: Yebo.

What comes out when he/she vomits?

Dr. Carlton: Kuphumani uma ehlanza?

Khekheleza: Ukudla nento eluhlaza engathi inyongo.

Did blood ever come out?

Dr. Carlton: Kuke kwaphuma igazi?

Khekheleza: Cha, alizange liphume.

Diarrhoea

Has he/she been passing loose stools?

Dr. Carlton: Siyamhabisa isisu? / Uyahhuda/ Uyakapakelwa isisu?

Khekheleza: Yebo,

Did blood ever come out?

Dr. Carlton: Kuke kwaphuma igazi?

Khekheleza: Cha, alizange liphume.

How many loose stools did he/she pass yesterday?

Dr. Carlton: Kangaki izolo?

Khekheleza: Kaningi.

How many times in number?

Dr. Carlton: Izihlandla ezingaki?

Khekheleza: Kwevile eshumini.

How many loose stools has he/she passed today?

Dr. Carlton: Kangaki namhlanje.

Khekheleza: Kathathu

Constipation

Has he/she not been passing stools?

Dr. Carlton: Ubophelene? Ubambekile? Ingabe usakaka?

Khekheleza: Cha,

When was the last time he/she passed stools?

Dr. Carlton: Ugcine nini ukukaka?

Khekheleza: Kuthangi.

Type of stools

How does the stool look like?

Dr. Carlton: Unjani umbala wamakaka? Ibukeka kanjani indle?

Khekheleza: Aphuzi futhi azihlambana ezincane.

Is there blood in the stools?

Dr. Carlton: Likhona igazi emakekeni? Ihambisana negazi indle?

Khekheleza: Cha,

Abdominal pain/ discomfort

Do you think they have abdominal pain?

Dr. Carlton: Uma ucabanga, unabo ubuhlungu esifubeni?

Khekheleza: Yebo, ngicabanga ukuthi uyasikeka lapha esiswini.

Why do you think he/she has abdominal pain?

Dr. Carlton: Ukucantshangiswa yini lokho.

Khekheleza: Ebusuku unokugoqana akhale ebamba isisu. / Ungitshele kanjalo.

Jaundice

Have you noticed that he/she has yellowing of the eyes and skin?

Dr. Carlton: Uke waxwaya ukuthi amehlo nesikhumba sakhe kuphuzi.

Khekheleza: Cha,

Genitourinary

Enuresis

Does he/she pass urine during sleep at night?

Dr. Carlton: Uyachama yini ebusuku uma elele, ukuchamela izingubo nombhede.

Khekheleza: Wagcini eneminyaka emithathu kepha useqalile futhi.

To distinguish between primary and secondary enuresis one has to ascertain whether there was a time when the child was dry at night.

Was there a time when they did not pass urine at night.

Dr. Carlton: Kukhona isikhathi lapho wayengazichameli?

Khekheleza: Yebo.

Dysuria

Does he/she have pain on passing urine?

Dr. Carlton: Unabo ubuhlungu uma echama.

Khekheleza: Angazi.

Frequency

Does he/she pass urine many times in a short space of time?

Dr. Carlton: Uchama kaningi esikhathini esifushane?

Khekheleza: Yebo, njalo nje ufuna ukuchama.

Polyuria

Is he/she passing large amounts of urine?

Dr. Carlton: Uchama umchamo omuningi yini?

Khekheleza: Yebo, uphuza abuye achama kakhulu.

Pyuria

Is there pus coming out when he/she passes urine?

Dr. Carlton: Kukhona ubovu oluphumayo uma echama?

Khekheleza: Bengingakaluboni.

Haematuria

Is there blood coming out when he/she passes urine?

Dr. Carlton: Kukhona igazi eliphumayo uma echama.

Khekheleza: Cha, alikho.

Vaginal discharge

Is there pus coming out of her private organ?

Dr. Carlton: Kukhona yini ubomvu oluphuma ngezansi.

Khekheleza: Cha, angikaluboni.

Is there blood coming out of her vagina?

Dr. Carlton: Kukhona yini igazi eliphumayo ngezansi?

Khekheleza: Yebo, elincane kodwa.

Penile/vaginal and testicular abnormalities

Does her vagina look normal?

Dr. Carlton: Ingabe isitho sakhe sangasese sibukeka sijwayelekile?

Khekheleza: Angazi.

Does his penis look normal?

Dr. Carlton: Ipipi/umfana/umpipi wakhe ubukeka ejwayelekile?

Khekheleza: Yebo.

Does he have two testicles?

Dr. Carlton: Ingabe unamaqanda amabili?

Khekheleza: Cha unelilodwa kwa-right.

Neuromuscular

Do you think your child is abnormal?

This question is rather insensitive it is better to ask . . .

Does your child look like other children?

Dr. Carlton: Ubukeka njengezinye izingane?

Khekheleza: Cha ngathi uhlukile.

In what way is he/she different?

Dr. Carlton: Uhluke kanjani?

Khekheleza: Unekhanda elincanyana kunezinye izingane.

Abnormal postures as part of a neuromuscular problem

Does he/she assume a sustained posture?

Dr. Carlton: Kukhona indlela ahlale eme ngayo angayiyeki.

Khekheleza: Yebo uhlale ebhekise ikhanda phezulu akavumi noma ulibuyisa.

Respiratory muscle weakness

Does he/she have difficulty breathing?

Dr. Carlton: Unayo inkinga nokuphefumula?

Khekheleza: Yebo, ngibona ngathi uphelelwa amadla uma ephefumula.

To elicit history about absence seizures

Does he/she appear to be absent minded at times?

Dr. Carlton: Kuyenzeka umbone sengathi akalalele/akekho/ andwaze?

Khekheleza: Yebo, kepha ubuya abuye emva kwemizuzwana.

Has he/she ever had a seizure?

Dr. Carlton: Wake wadlikiza/wadikiza?

Khekheleza: Yebo, wayenemfiva esemuncane.

Does he/she have seizure sickness?

Dr. Carlton: Unesifo sokudlikiza?

Dr. Carlton: Kuyamhlupha yini ukudlikiza njalo? Une-ephilephsi

Khekheleza: Cha.

Does he/she get tired too quickly, compared to other children?

Dr. Carlton: Uyashesa yini ukukhathala kunezinye izingane.

Khekheleza: Hhayi, uyadlala kuze kuphele.

Endocrine

Does he/she appear not to be growing well?

Dr. Carlton: Ngokubona kwakho ukhula kahle.

Khekheleza: Yebo.

Does he/she appear to be growing too fast?

Dr. Carlton: Ngokubona kwakho, ukhula ngokushesha yini?

Khekheleza: Cha, ukhula kahle nje.

Does he/she drink a lot more that he/she should?

Dr. Carlton: Uphuza amanzi ngokweqile yini kunokujwayelekile?

Khekheleza: Yebo, sikhashana nje useyophuza amanzi.

Does he/she eat more than you think he/she should?

Dr. Carlton: Udla kakhulu yini kunokujwayelekile?

Khekheleza: Cha, udla kahle.

Have you noticed any swelling on the neck?

Dr. Carlton: Uke waxwaya ukudumba noma ukuvuvuka entanyeni?

Khekheleza: Cha, akunalutho.

General

Weight loss

Do you think that he/she is losing weight?

Dr. Carlton: Uyancipha yini emzimbeni?

Khekheleza: Yebo, ngibona sengathi unciphile impela.

Abnormal weight gain

Do you think that he/she is gaining too much weight?

Dr. Carlton: Ukhuluphala ngokushesha kakhulu yini?

OR

Dr. Carlton: Awucabangi ukuthi unone kakhulu?

Khekheleza: Hhayi, wondleke kahle nje.

Time of pubescence

At was age did you notice puberty?

Dr. Carlton: Ubeneminyaka emingaki mhla ubona izimpawu zokuthomba?

Khekheleza: Ubeneminyaka engu—12.

Pattern of pubescence

Do you think that he/she went through purberty the normal way?

Dr. Carlton: Ucabanga ukuthi uthomba kahle/ngokujwayelekile?

Khekheleza: Yebo, akukho engikuxwayayo.

Past medical history

The mother's medical history

Mothers medical and obstetric history

Does the mother have any medical problems?

Dr. Carlton: Ingabe umama wontwana unako lo kugula okulandelayo?

In case where the mother is present to give the history

Do you any of the following illnesses?

Dr. Carlton: Unako lo kugula okulandelayo?

A better question to ask is whether they have been informed in a previous occasion about the illnesses and or are taking treatment for the illness because there tends to be a lot of misunderstanding about illness and disease between the patients and doctors. As an example some patients believe that a headache equates to high blood pressure and will actually say they have increased blood pressure because of the headache. There are various other symptoms that patients tend to attribute disease to where a formal diagnosis has yet to be made.

Hypertension or high blood pressure?

Dr. Carlton: I—BP?

Do you take medication for BP/hypertension?

Dr. Carlton: Uyawathatha/ Uyawadla amaphilisi e-BP?

Diabetes/ Sugar disease

Dr. Carlton: I—diabetes/ushukela?

Do you take medication for diabetes/sugar?

Dr. Carlton: Uyawathatha/ Uyawadla amaphilisi e-diabetes?

Do you use injections for diabetes/sugar disease?

Dr. Carlton: Uyayisebenzisa imijovo ye-diabetes/ushukela?

Tuberculosis

Dr. Carlton: I-TB/ isifuba se-TB?

Do you take medication for TB?

Dr. Carlton: Uyawathatha/ Uyawadla amaphilisi e-TB?

Previous TB

Have you ever had TB before?

Dr. Carlton: Wake waba ne-TB?

When?

Dr. Carlton: Kwakunini?

TB exposure (especially for children)

Is there anyone with TB at home?

Dr. Carlton: Ukhona one-TB ekhaya?

Epilepsy

Do you have epilepsy/fitting disease/seizure disease?

Dr. Carlton: Unayo i-epilepsy/isifo sokudikiza/isifo sokudlikiza?

Do you take medication for epilepsy/ seizure disease?

Dr. Carlton: Uyawathatha/ Uyawadla amaphilisi e-epilepsy/ esifo sokudlikiza?

Cardiac disease

Do you have cardiac disease?

Dr. Carlton: Isifo senhliziyo?

Do you take medication for cardiac disease?

Dr. Carlton: Uyawathatha/ Uyawadla amaphilisi esifo senhliziyo?

Asthma

Dr. Carlton: I—asthma?

Do you take medication for asthma?

Dr. Carlton: Uyawathatha/ Uyawadla amaphilisi e-BP?

Do you have or use pumps for asthma?

Dr. Carlton: Unazo noma uyazisebenzisa izifutho ze-asthma.

Renal disease

Dr. Carlton: Isifo sezinso?

Do you take medication for BP/hypertension?

Dr. Carlton: Uyawathatha/ Uyawadla amaphilisi e-BP?

HIV/AIDS

Dr. Carlton: I-HIV/intsholongwane?

Do you take medication for HIV?

Dr. Carlton: Uyawathatha/ Uyawadla amaphilisi e-HIV?

OR

Is the mother on ARV's.

Dr. Carlton: Umama uyawadla yini ama-ARV's

If not was the prevention of mother to child transmission utilized?

Dr. Carlton: Uma engawadli kwenziwa yini ukuthi kuvikelwe ukudlulisela intsholongwana emntwaneni?

Is the mother taking any chronic medications?

Dr. Carlton: Akhona yini amaphilisi noma umuthi umama aphila ngokuwadla?

Did the mother have any illnesses in the antenatal period?

Dr. Carlton: Kukhona yini ukugula okuke kwahlupha umama ngenkathi esakhulelwe?

Vaginal discharge

Did the mother have vaginal discharge in pregnancy?

Dr. Carlton: Ingabe kwaba khona okuphumayo ngezansi kumama ngesikhathi esakhulelwe?

Did the mother have any illnesses in the peripartum period?

Dr. Carlton: Kwaba khona ukugula okwahlupha umama ngenkathi eseduze kokubelethwa komntwana?

Did the mother have any illnesses in the post partum period?

Dr. Carlton: Kwaba khona ukugula okuhlupha umama ngesikhathi kuqedwa kubelethwa umntwana?

Birth history

Was the birth normal or assisted?

Dr. Carlton: Ingabe umntwana wabelethwa kahle noma ngokusizwa?

Was the birth by an operation/ caesarian section?

Dr. Carlton: Umntwana wabelethwa ngokusikwa/ nge-operation/ i-caesarian section?

Was the birth at term i.e. 9 months or 37 weeks? Before i.e. < 36 weeks? or After i.e. >39 weeks?

Dr. Carlton: Ingabe umntwana wabelethwa ngesikhathi; izinyanga ezingu-9? noma singakafiki; ngaphambi kwezinyanga ezingu-8? Noma sesedlule; izinyanga ezingu-10 sezedlule.

Were there any problems with the child that necessitated a longer stay after birth?

Dr. Carlton: Zaba khona izinkinga ezenza ukuthi kudingeke ukuthi umntwana ahlale esibhedlela ngesikhathi esebelethiwe?

Pnemonia

Did the child have pneumonia after birth?

Dr. Carlton: Umntwana waba nayo yini i-pneumonia ngesikhathi eqeda ukubelethwa?

Jaundice

Dr. Carlton: Umntwana waba nayo yini i-jaundice ngesikhathi eqeda ukubelethwa?

OR

Dr. Carlton: Umntwana waba nalo yini ijondisi ngesikhathi eqeda ukubelethwa?

OR

Did the child have yellowing of the eyes and skin (jaundice) after birth?

Dr. Carlton: Umntwana waba nako yini ukuba phuzi kwamehlo nesikhumba mhla eqeda ukubelethwa?

Family history

Pregnancy planned or unplanned

Dr. Carlton: Ingabe kwakuhleliwe yini ukuzethwala kukamama?

Did the mother plan to fall pregnant?

Dr. Carlton: Umama wabe ezilungiselele ukuzethwala?

Couple married or not?

Dr. Carlton: Ingabe abazali bomntwana basemshadweni yini?

Is the mother of the child married to the father of the child.

Dr. Carlton: Ingabe umama womntwana umshadile yini ubaba womntwana?

Living arrangement

Who lives with the child?

Dr. Carlton: Umntwana uhlala nobani?

Child care

Who looks after the child during the day?

Dr. Carlton: Umntwana unakekelwa ngubani emini?

Consanguinity

Are the mother and father closely related?

Dr. Carlton: Ingabe umama nobaba womntwana bahlobene?

Siblings

Where are the brothers and sisters of the child?

Dr. Carlton: Bakuphi abafowabo kanye nodadewabo bomntwana?

How old are they?

Dr. Carlton: Baneminyaka emingaki?

Do they have any illnesses?

Dr. Carlton: Kukhona ukugula okubahluphayo?

Developmental history

The gross and fine motor development

Raising the head

At what age (in months) was the child noticed to be able to raise the head when lying on the belly?

Dr. Carlton: Wabe engakanani (ngezinyanga) umntwana ngesikhathi esekwazi ukuvusa ikhanda uma elele ngesisu?

Rolling over

At what age was the child able to roll over from a prone position to a supine position (lying with the belly to lying with the back)?

Dr. Carlton: Wabe engakanani umntwana ngesikhathi kubonakala ukuthi uyakwazi ukuphenduka ekulaneni ngesisu alale ngomhlane?

Sitting unassisted

At what age was the child noticed to be able to sit alone.

Dr. Carlton: Wabe engakanani umntwana ngesikhathi kubonakala ukuthi uyakhona ukuzihlalela yedwa?

Pulling up to stand

At what age was the child noticed to be able to pull to stand with objects?

Dr. Carlton: Wabe engakanani umntwana ngesikhathi kubonakala ukuthi uyakwazi ukudonsa izinto ame ngazo?

Walking unassisted

At what age was the child noticed to be able to walk alone (unassisted)

Dr. Carlton: Wabe engakanani umntwana ngesikhathi kubonakala ukuthi useyacathuza?

Grasping and releasing

At what age was the child noticed to be able to release objects when grasped with the whole hand?

Dr. Carlton: Wabe engakanani umntwana ngesikhathi kubonakala ukuthi uyakwazi ukudedela izinto abekade ezibambe ngezadla engaphuciwe?

Grasping with fingers
At what age was the child noticed to be able to hold objects using fingers as opposed to using the whole hand
Dr. Carlton: Wabe engakanani umntwana ngesikhathi kubonakala ukuthi uyakwazi ukubamba izinto ngeminwe kunokubamba ngesandla sonke?

Mental development and language
Babbling sounds
At what age was the child noticed to be able to make babbling sounds?
Dr. Carlton: Wabe engakanani umntwana ngesikhathi kubonakala ukuthi usekwazi ukwenza imisindo yokubhibhidla?

Saying meaningful words
At what age was the child noticed to be able to say a few audible words?
Dr. Carlton: Wabe engakanani umntwana ngesikhathi kubonakala ukuthi useyakwazi ukusho amagama azwakalayo?

Speaking in sentences
At what age was the child noticed to be able to speak in sentences?
Dr. Carlton: Wabe engakanani umntwana ngesikhathi kubonakala ukuthi usekwazi ukukhuluma imisho?

Stranger anxiety
At what age was the child noticed to be able to be less scared of strangers?
Dr. Carlton: Wabe engakanani umntwana ngesikhathi kubonakala ukuthi ukasababi abantu angabazi?

Continence

How old was the child noticed to be dry at night?

Dr. Carlton: Wabe engakanani umntwana ngesikhathi kubonakala ukuthi akazichameli ebusuku?

If the child has a problem of bed wetting (nocturnal enuresis) one needs to ascertain if it is primary or secondary.

Has there ever been a time when the child was dry at night for more than 5 nights in a week.

Dr. Carlton: Kwake kwaba khona isikhathi lapho umntwana wake wahlala engazichameli ebusuku izinsuku ezinhlanu evikini?

School grades

How is the child performing at school?

Dr. Carlton: Unjani umntwana esikoleni?

Vaccinations/ Immunizations

Did the child receive all their immunizations?

Dr. Carlton: Ingabe umntwana ugomile/ uhlabile ngokuphelele?

The Road to Health Chart

Did you bring the road to health chart (child clinic chart) with you?

Dr. Carlton: Uliphathile ikhadi lomntwana lase-clinic?

After the completion of history taking

Conclusion of History Taking

Thank the patient for having participated in answering your questions.
Dr. Carlton: Ngiyabonga

Mention that you would then like to do an examination.
Dr. Carlton: Manje ngicela ukukuhlola umzimba.

- Being polite will allow the patient to be cooperative through the examination.
- The help you shall acquire is to get the patient to assume positions that you can find suitable to carry out the examination.
- The way to convey statements is easier to give as orders but it shall be made polite by adding a "please" before the statements. In the beginning you may choose to omit the please but as you get used to talking you may reinstal it as appropriate as it is inappropriate to have it all the time.
- Please.

Dr. Carlton: Ngiyakucela.

S AY IT PRIOR to all statements made if you mean to be polite. Saying it after the statements is just as good. We shall have it in brackets as it is an optional expression to make.

- I would like to examine your body.

Dr. Carlton: Ngithanda ukukuhlola umzimba.

- Asking the patent to sit down.

Dr. Carlton: (Ngiyakucela). Hlala phansi.

OR

Dr. Carlton: Ngicela uhlale phansi.

Stand up.

Dr. Carlton: Sukuma.

Sit up.

Dr. Carlton: Vuka/ Vuka uhlale.

- Asking the patient to sit or lie down

Please sit on the bed.

Dr. Carlton: (Ngiyakucela). Hlala embhedeni.

Please lie on the bed.

Dr. Carlton: (Ngiyakucela). Lala embhedeni.

Khekheleza: Ngilale embhedeni?

If the patient repeats what you have just said reply by saying yes (yebo) and they shall do it.

- Asking to see the patient's hands.

Dr. Carlton: Ngicela ukubona izandla zakho.

- Asking to see the patient's eyes:

Dr. Carlton: Ngicela ukukubona amehlo.

- Asking to see the patient's feet.

Dr. Carlton: Ngicela ukukubona izinyawo.

Please take off your shoes and socks.

Dr. Carlton: (Ngiyakucela). Khumula izicathulo namasokisi.

VITALS SIGNS

- Blood Pressure.

Dr. Carlton: Ngicela ukukala i-blood pressure.

Give your right arm.

Dr. Carlton: Ngiphe ingalo yangakwesokudla.

Left arm—Ingalo yesinxele.
You may also use:
Left arm—Ingalo yakwa-left
Right arm—Ingalo yakwa-right

Temperature

Dr. Carlton: Ngicela ukukala izinga lokushisa.

I shall put the thermometer in your armpit for 3 minutes.

Dr. Carlton: Ngizobeka i-thermometer ekhwapheni imizuzu emithathu.

I shall put the thermometer under your tongue for 3 minutes.

Dr. Carlton: Ngizobeka i-thermometer ngaphansi kolimi imizuzu emithathu.

The pulse and respiratory rate shall be done without alerting the patient.

- At this point you would have made an assessment of the general appearance and noted other strikingly obvious clinical features.

- Based on the history, a system has been chosen to base the rest of the examination.

Inspection of the head and neck:

- Please look to the right.

Dr. Carlton: (Ngiyakucela). Bheka ngakwesokudla/ kwa-right?

- to the left—ngakwesokunxele/ kwa-left

- Please look up.

Dr. Carlton: (Ngiyakucela). Bheka phezulu.

- down—phansi

- I would like to look at the back of your head.

Dr. Carlton: Ngithanda ukukubheka esiphundu/ ekhanda ngemuva.

- Please swallow.

Dr. Carlton: (Ngiyakucela). Gwinya.

- Put your ear on your shoulder.

Dr. Carlton: Beka indlebe ehlombe.

SYSTEMIC EXAMINATION

I N THE FOLLOWING examples of examination an occasional short history is given; this is to aid with further questioning that may not have been elicited during general history which is more specific to the system that is to be examined.

THE HEAD AND NECK

EAR, NOSE AND THROAT FOCUSSED HISTORY.

Ear

Earache:
I have pain on my left ear.
Khekheleza: Indlebe yami yakwa-left ibuhlungu.

Ear discharge:
I have pus coming out of my right ear.
Khekheleza: Indlebe yami iphuma ubomvu.

Other forms of ear discharges
Blood—igazi
Serous (clear) fluid—uketshezi olucwebile.
You are more likely to hear about water than this.
Water—amanzi

I have a bead (or any other foreign body) in my ear.
Khekheleza: Nginobuhlalu endlebeni.

Nose:

My nose is blocked.
Khekheleza: Ngicinene.

I have a nose bleed. (this is likely to be an observation to make before the patient tells you)
Khekheleza: Nginomongoziya/ ngopha ekhaleni.

I have some clear fluid dripping from my nose.
Khekheleza: Kunoketshezi olucwebile oluphuma amakhaleni.

My nose is broken.
Khekheleza: Ikhala lami liphukile.

Throat:

Throat pain?
Dr. Carlton: Unabo ubuhlungu emphinjeni?
Khekheleza: Yebo.

Do you have pain on swallowing.
Dr. Carlton: Kubuhlungu uma ugwinya?
Khekheleza: Yebo uma ngidla ukudla okomile.

Coughing?
Dr. Carlton: Uyakhwehlela?

Khekheleza: Yebo

Examination

At this point the patient shall be seated.
Ears:
I would like to look at your ear.
Dr. Carlton: Ngithanda ukukubheka endlebeni.

I am going to use this instrument/ otoscope. (shows the patient the instrument)
Dr. Carlton: Ngizosebenzisa lo mshini/ i-otoscope.

It shall not be painful.
Dr. Carlton: Angeke kube buhlungu.
OR
Dr. Carlton: Akubuhlungu

Tell me if it is uncomfortable/ painful.
Dr. Carlton: Ungazise uma kubuhlungu.

Your ear is dirty and I shall remove the dirt.
Dr. Carlton: Indlebe yakho ingcolile. Ngizokhipha udoti.

Nose:

I would like to look into your nose.
Dr. Carlton: Ngithanda ukukubheka emakhaleni.

I shall use this instrument (show instrument).
Dr. Carlton: Ngizosebenzisa loku.

Clean your nose. (Give a tissue)
Dr. Carlton: Khipha amafinyila/ finya.

Breathe through the nose.
Dr. Carlton: Phefumula ngamakhala.

Close your mouth.
Dr. Carlton: Vala umlomo.

Open your mouth.
Dr. Carlton: Vula umlomo.

Breathe though the mouth.
Dr. Carlton: Phefumula ngomlomo.

The Throat:

I would like to look into your throat.
Dr. Carlton: Ngithanda ukubheka emphinjeni.

Please. Open your mouth.
Dr. Carlton: (Ngiyakucela). Vula umlomo.
OR
Dr. Carlton: Ngicela uvule umlomo.

Open your moth wider.
Dr. Carlton: Vula umlomo kakhulu.

Stick out (protrude) your tongue.
Dr. Carlton: Khipha ulimi.

Move your tongue up.
Dr. Carlton: Yisa ulimi phezulu.

Move your tongue down
Dr. Carlton: Yisa ulimi phansi.

Say AAH.
Dr. Carlton: Ithi/ thani AAH.

If you would like to demonstrate
Do like this (then show).
Dr. Carlton: Yenza kanje.
(Demonstrating is best)

Musculoskeletal Examination of the Neck

History—already established
Neck pain—Ubuhlungu bentamo

Pain on turning head—Ubuhlungu uma kuphendulwa ikhanda

A mass on the neck.—Ukuvuvuka, noma ilunda entanyeni.

The history may be of a neurological lesion of the upper limbs that warrant
examination of the cervical spine.

Remember to Look, Feel and Move.
I—LOOK
This needs to be done to an adequately exposed patient.
Ask the patient to take off their upper clothing.

Please take off your upper clothing from the waist upwards.

Dr. Carlton: Ngicela ukhumule izingubo kusuka okhalweni kuya phezulu.

Look for abnormalities, e.g. abnormal posture.

II—FEEL

You touch and feel the bony prominences and any skeletal abnormalities and ask about pain/ and tenderness.

Another position that the patient may need to assume is prone with a pillow under the shoulder to slightly flex the neck.

Please could you lie on the bed facing down.

Dr. Carlton: Ngicela ulale embhedeni ubheke phansi

Put a pillow under your shoulders.

Dr. Carlton: Ubeke umqamelo ngaphansi kwamahlombe.

III—MOVE

Firstly its passive movements then active movement.

Active movements

Neck flexion and extension.

Please put your chin on your chest.

Dr. Carlton: Beka isilevu esifubeni.

Please look up as much as you can.

Dr. Carlton: Bheka phezulu kuze kufike lapho ugcina khona.

Lateral flexion.

Please put your ear on your shoulder without lifting the shoulder.

Dr. Carlton: Beka indlebe ehlombe ungaliphakamisi ihlombe.

This side as well.
Dr. Carlton: Nangapha.

Do it on the other side as well.
Dr. Carlton: Yenza futhi kolunye uhlangothi.

Neck rotation
Look to the left.
Dr. Carlton: Bheka kwa-left.

Then look to the right.
Dr. Carlton: Bese ubheka kwa-right.

If you would like to demonstrate.
Do like this (then show).
Dr. Carlton: Yenza kanje.
(Demonstrating is best)

Passive Movements
Ask the patient to relax the neck and inform them that you are going to be moving it for them.
Please relax your neck.
Dr. Carlton: Ngicela uthambise intamo.

I am going to be moving your neck for you.
Dr. Carlton: Ngizoyinyakazisa mina.

Tell me if you are feeling pain.
Dr. Carlton: Ungitshele uma kubuhlungu.
OR ask: Is it painful? (While doing the passive movements).

Dr. Carlton: Kubuhlungu?
Khekheleza: Eish (exclaiming with pain)!!!

You then move the joints noting resistance to movement, range of motion and the patients' face for pain.

EXAMINATION OF THE CHEST

EXPOSURE AND POSITIONING

Please take off your upper clothing from the waist upwards.
Dr. Carlton: Ngicela ukhumule izingubo kusuka okhalweni kuya phezulu.

Please take off your jacket &/ jersey/ shirt/ t-shirt/ vest.
Dr. Carlton: Ngicela ukhumule i-jacket noma i-jersey/ i-shirt/ i-t-shirt/ i-vest.

See the obvious e.g. wasting, asymmetry, scars etc.

Sit on the bed with your legs hanging on the side.
Dr. Carlton: Hlala embhedeni ulengise izinyawo.

You then inspect the patient for any skin or skeletal abnormalities. Ask about such abnormalities.
(take note of symmetry, intercostal drain scars, rashes, marks from scratching, chest hyper-inflation, pigeon chest, barrel chest, funnel chest, kyphoscoliosis etc.)

What is this?
Dr. Carlton: Yini le?
Khekheleza: Isibazi

Scar—isibazi

When did you get this scar?
Dr. Carlton: Walimala nini lapha?
Khekheleza: Ngo 2000.

When did you have a rash?
Dr. Carlton: Ube nayo nini i-rash?
Khekheleza: Ngisasemncane.

EXAMINATION OF THE AXILLA

I—Inspection
I would like to look at your underarms.
Dr. Carlton: Ngicela ukukubheka emakhwapheni.

Lift your arms/hands.
Dr. Carlton: Phakamisa izingalo/izandla.

II—Palpation (position the patient correctly)
I would like to feel for glands in your underarms.
Dr. Carlton: Ngicela ukuzwa ukuthi akukho amalunda emakhwapheni.

Please lift your arms (demonstrate).
Dr. Carlton: Ngicela uphakamise izingalo.

Lift your arms. (put your hand in position)
Dr. Carlton: Phakamisa izingalo.

Bring your arms down.
Dr. Carlton: Yehlisa izingalo.

THE RESPITATORY SYSTEM

I—Inspection
Having looked for scars and skeletal abnormalities now look at the chest movements with respiration; costal recessions, use of accessory respiratory muscles and asymmetry in chest movements. Ask the patient to take deep breaths. This makes things more well-defined.

Please could you breathe in and out deeply?
Dr. Carlton: Ngicela uphefumulele phuzulu udonse uphinde ukhiphe umoya.

II—Palpation
The trachea, pain over the ribs, chest expansion, vocal fremitus, apex beat etc.
Please say ninety-nine.
Dr. Carlton: Dr. Carlton: Ngicela uthi ninety-nine.

Again.—Futhi.

III—Percusion
All areas, apices, over the clavicles and underarms. Remember liver and cardiac dullness.

IV—Auscultation

Vocal resonance—Important to confirm vocal fremitus.

Please say ninety-nine.

Dr. Carlton: Ngicela uthi ninety-nine.

Again.—Futhi.

Breath sounds, added sounds.

Please could you breathe deeply in and out with your mouth open.

Dr. Carlton: Ngicela uphefumulele phezulu, udonse uphinde ukhiphe umoya uvule umlomo.

Or demonstrate

Please breathe like this. (Mouth open or closed taking deep breaths).

Dr. Carlton: Ngicela uphefumule kanje.

Other parts of the examination

The Pemberton's Sign

Please lift your arms and keep them up.

Dr. Carlton: Ngicela uphakamise izingalo uzimise phezulu.

Put them down.

Dr. Carlton: Zehlise.

If you would like to demonstrate.

Do like this (then show).

Dr. Carlton: Yenza kanje.

(Demonstrating is best)

EXAMINATION OF THE BREASTS

Exposure and Positioning
I would like to examine your breasts.
Dr. Carlton: Ngithanda ukuhlola amabele.

Please could you take off your bra (brassiere).
Dr. Carlton: Ngicela ukhumule u-bra (brassiere).

For arm positioning demonstrate to the patient.
Dr. Carlton: Beka ingalo kanje.

Inspection
While the patient is upright inspect the breasts for symmetry and any skin abnormalities. Ask them to lift their arms for you to inspect the breasts.

Please lift up your arms.
Dr. Carlton: Ngicela uphakamise izingalo.

Please press on your hips [like this]. (demonstrate)
Dr. Carlton: Ngicela ucindezele okhalweni [kanje].
Note skin abnormalities, areola changes, and asymmetry also ask about it.

Palpation
Please lay on the bed facing up.
Dr. Carlton: Ngicela ulale embhedeni ubheke phezulu.

Continue inspection and start palpation.
Ask about tenderness before you start and while you are palpating.
Pain on the breasts.

Dr. Carlton: Unabo ubuhlungu emabeleni?
Khekheleza: Buba khona uma ngizoya esikhathini.

Where, point?
Dr. Carlton: Kuphi, khomba?
OR while palpating ask . . .
Is it painful?
Dr. Carlton: Kubuhlungu?

Feel for lumps, and any other abnormalities, ask about them.
Remember to palpate the axillary tail, the nipple-areola complex and try to express milk or a discharge as guided by the history.
Evaluate lumps when found.
Examine the axilla as well.

The armpits as well.
Dr. Carlton: Namakhwapha.

THE CARDIOVASCULAR EXAMINATION (THE PRAECORDIUM)

EXPSOSURE AND POSITIONING

The general examination would have been done as per body site involved, peripheral pulses checked and assessed, blood pressure measured
The patient must have their upper bodies undressed.

Please take off your upper clothing from the waist upwards.
Dr. Carlton: Ngicela ukhumule izingubo kusuka okhalweni kuya phezulu.

Having done the general examination you can adjust the bed and ask the patient to lie down.

Please lie on the bed facing up.
Dr. Carlton: Ngicela ulale embhedeni ubheke phezulu

Please put your arms on your sides.
Dr. Carlton: Ngicela ubeke izingalo eceleni kwakho.

I—Inspection

To ask the patient to seat up for you to adjust the bed to horizontal or any other angle.
Please seat up.
Dr. Carlton: Ngicela uvuke uhlale.

Please lay down again.
Dr. Carlton: Ngicela ulale futhi.

The jugular venous pressure. With the patient lying on the bed with the head elevated to 45 degrees.
Please look to the left.
Dr. Carlton: Ngicela ubheke kwa-left.

Remember to do the hepatojugular reflex, assess the waveforms and palpate the neck area as part of the evaluation

General, for skeletal abnormalities and skin lesions
The praecordium, inspect for scars and ask what caused them if it was not revealed during the history taking.

The apex beat can be visible on thin individuals.

II—Palpation

I am to touch and feel your heart on the chest.

Dr. Carlton: Ngizokuthinta esifubeni ukuze ngizwe inhliziyo.

Apex beat, palpable pulmonary tap, the parasternal heave must all be felt and described if palpable.

III—Percussion

Just percuss

IV—Auscultation

Now I am going to listen on your chest for your heart.

Dr. Carlton: Manje ngizolalela esifubeni kuze ngizwe inhliziyo.

Auscultate over all areas and on the axilla and neck if needed. Do not forget the lung bases.

Dynamic auscultation.

Breathe in deeply and hold your breath.

Dr. Carlton: Donsa umoya bese uma ukuphefumula.

Breathe out deeply and hold your breath.

Dr. Carlton: Khipha umoya bese uma ukuphefumula.

(The periods of breathholding should not be prolonged)

Please sleep on your left hand side.

Dr. Carlton: Ngicela ulale ngecala lakwa-left.

Please wake up and lean forward.
Dr. Carlton: Ngicela uvuke bese ugobela ngaphambili.

You may ask the patient to squat. (this is not usually done)
Squat—Qoshama

You may ask the patient sit up so you can adjust the examination couch e.g. have the patient lying flat.

Valsava manoeuvre
Please close your nose with your fingers. (demonstrate)
Dr. Carlton: Ngicela uvale amakhala uwacindizele ngeminnwe.
THEN
Close your mouth and push out the air so as to pop your ears.
Dr. Carlton: Uvale umlomo bese ufutha umoya kuze kucinane izindlebe.

EXAMINATION OF THE ABDOMEN

EXPOSURE AND POSITIONING
The patient should ideally be exposed from the nipples to the knees for a proper abdominal examination.
After having done the general examination

Please could you expose your stomach area (abdomen) from the nipples down to your knees? (You may need a chaperone for this)
Dr. Carlton: Ngicela ukhumule uveze isisu kusukela ngaphansi kwamabele (izibele) kuya emadolweni.

Male breasts—Izibele

This is usually not the case so just ask the patient to lift up their upper clothing and lower their lower clothing to the waist appropriately.

I would like to examine your abdomen.
Dr. Carlton: Ngithanda ukukuhlola esiswini.

Please could you lift up your clothes to expose your abdomen?
Dr. Carlton: Ngicela uphakamise izingubo ukuze uveze isisu

Please undo (loosen) your belt?
Dr. Carlton: Ngicela uqhaqhe (uxegise) ibhande.

Please lower your trouser/ skirt?
Dr. Carlton: Ngicela wehlise ibhulukwe/ isiketi.

The patient should be in a supine position with a pillow under their heads and their arms on their sides
Please lie on the bed facing up?
Dr. Carlton: Ngicela ulale embhedeni ubheke phezulu.

Please put your arms on your sides?
Dr. Carlton: Ngicela ubeke izingalo eceleni kwakho.

I—Inspection
With the patient lying on a supine position with an appropriately exposed abdomen inspect for symmetry, scars, distension, veins, pulsations, movements with respiration (you may have to view this from the side), skin lesions etc.

II—Palpation

Before touching ask if there is pain.

Where is it painful?

Dr. Carlton: Kubuhlungu kuphi?

Point?

Dr. Carlton: Khomba?

OR while palpating ask

Is it painful?

Dr. Carlton: Kubuhlungu?

II—Palpation

If the abdomen is tense ask the patient to bend their knees to relax the abdominal muscles.

Please could you bend your knee a little?

Dr. Carlton: Ngicela ugobise amadolo kancane.

Begin with light palpation from a point furthest from the pain. Be looking at the patient's face to see if you are eliciting tenderness.

Then proceed to deep palpation feeling for masses and tenderness, if a mass is found it must be localised and described fully.

Other examination procedures like rebound tenderness should not be left out.

If you wish to distinguish an abdominal wall mass from the intra-abdominal mass you may ask the supine patient to lift their legs/ head to tense the abdominal wall.

Please lift your head.

Dr. Carlton: Ngicela uphakamise ikhanda.

OR

Please lift your legs straight up just a bit.

Dr. Carlton: Ngicela uphakamise imilenze kancane uyiqondisile.

The palpation of the inguinal lymph nodes shall be discussed in the next section (examination of the pelvis)

Palpation for an enlarged spleen

Starting from the right / left iliac fossa with the radial edge of the palm parallel to the left sub costal line palpate asking the patient to breathe in and out. Remember to have your other hand over the patients left lower ribs to have the skin less tense which may aid in easier detection of the spleen.

Please breathe deeply in and out.

Dr. Carlton: Ngicela uphefumulele phezulu udonse uphinde ukhiphe umoya.

Again.—Futhi.

Be advancing closer to the left sub costal line as the patient repeats the breathing until you can feel the splenic edge hitting your finger on patient's inspiration.

Ask the patient to lie on the right hand side. This also helps with the detection of the spleen.

Please lie on your right.

Dr. Carlton: Ngicela ulale ngecala lakwa-right.

Then the palpation asking the patient to breathe deeply in and out as has been done.

Palpation of the kidneys

This is called ballotment.

On a supine patient have the palmer part of your fingers in the space between the lowest ribs and the iliac bones. Do the balloting movements (up and down pressure) as the patient breathes deeply.

Please breathe deeply in and out.

Dr. Carlton: Ngicela uphefumulele phezulu udonse uphinde ukhiphe umoya.

Again.—Futhi.

Palpation for an enlarged liver

Starting from the right iliac fossa with the radial edge of the palm parallel to the right sub costal line palpate asking the patient to breathe in and out.

Please breathe deeply in and out.

Dr. Carlton: Ngicela uphefumulele phezulu udonse uphinde ukhiphe umoya.

Again.—Futhi.

Be moving closer (intervals of 1-2 cm) to the costal line as the patient repeats the breathing until you can feel the liver edge hitting your hand on patient's inspiration.

The palpation of the gall bladder can be carried out simultaneously.

III—Percussion

Remember to percuss all areas, for tenderness, to map out masses and the work out liver span at mid clavicular line on the right hand side.

The splenic enlargement can be excluded by percussing the lower left intercostal spaces.

IV—Ausculatation

Over the areas that matter (for the abdominal aorta, liver, and renal arteries) and as guided by the history and other examination findings.

EXAMINATION OF THORACOLUMBER SPINE MUSCULOSKELETAL EXAMINATION

The history will suggest the need for this part of the examination.

I—Look

Exposure and positioning

The patient should be without upper body clothing and should be standing.

Please take off your upper clothing from the waist upwards.

Dr. Carlton: Ngicela ukhumule izingubo kusuka okhalweni kuya phezulu.

Observing the patients as they undress is of value to see if they are having any difficulties or assuming any unusual postures.

Look for symmetry, kyphosis, scoliosis, exaggerated lordosis visible muscular spasms, other skin and skeletal abnormalities.

Ask the patient to walk in the room, turn and walk the other way. This is to see any abnormalities in gait.

Please walk over there (point) and back.

Dr. Carlton: Ngicela uhambe uyojika lapha uphinde ubuye.

II—FEEL

Let the patient know that you shall touch their backs and ribs and ask them to relax.

I am going to touch your back and ribs to see if they are alright.

Dr. Carlton: Ngizokuthinta eqolo nezimbambo ukuze ngizwe ukuthi zilungile.

Khekheleza: Kulungile

Let me know if you feel pain.

Dr. Carlton: Ungazise uma uzwa ubuhlungu.

III—MOVE

Active movements

Flexion and extension

Please could you bend and touch your toes.

Dr. Carlton: Ngicela ugobe uthinte izinzwane.

Please could you bend backwards as much as you can? (May need to demonstrate)

Dr. Carlton: Ngicela uzilule/ uqethuke uze ufike la ugcina khona.

Ensure the patient does not fall for the latter motion. To demonstrate:

Do like this (demonstrate).

Dr. Carlton: Yenza kanje.

If you use a tape measure to measure the patients while bending

I am going to measure with a tape to see how far you bend.

Dr. Carlton: Ngizokala nge-tape ukuze ngibone ukuthi ugoba kangakanani.

Lateral Flexion

Please run your hand down the side of you leg and bend sideways.

Dr. Carlton: Ngicela uhambise isandla sakho emlenzeni ugobele ngaseceleni.

To the left.
Dr. Carlton: Ngakwa-left

To the right.
Dr. Carlton: Ngakwa-right
OR alternatively do one side and say
This side as well.
Dr. Carlton: Nangapha.

Rotation
The patient may have to sit down to stabilise the pelvis and you need to ask them to fold their arms so the motion is not exaggerated by arm movements.

I am going to stabilise your hip bones while you do the following movements. (then stabilise the pelvis)
Dr. Carlton: Ngizokubamba okhalweni uma wenza leminyakazo elandelayo.
OR Sit on the bed.
Dr. Carlton: Hlale embhedeni.

Please fold your arms like this. (demonstrate).
Dr. Carlton: Ngicela usonge izingalo kanje.

Please turn your body to the right then to the left.
Dr. Carlton: Ngicela ujikise umzimba uwubhekise kwa-right bese ubheka kwa-left.

For Passive movements ask the patient to relax and you shall move them.
Please relax I shall move your joints.

Dr. Carlton: Ngicela uthambise umzimba ngizokunyakazisa mina ama-joints.

EXAMINATION OF THE PELVIS AND THE PERINEUM

The Anorectal Examination (Digital Rectum Examination)

Male health care workers require a chaperone when perfoming the procedure on female patients. Have gloves and tissue/gauze handy.
Inform the patient for the need for this examination; tell patients how you need for them to position themselves.

I would like to check your back passage.
Dr. Carlton: Ngithanda ukuhlola imbobo yangemuva.
OR
Dr. Carlton: Ngicela ukuhlola imbobo yamakaka.
OR
I would like to check your anus (shit-whole).—Ngithanda ukukuhlola "umdidi"/ "indunu"

To ask the patient to take off their lower clothing:
Please could you take off your lower clothing?
Dr. Carlton: Ngicela ukhumule izingubo zangezansi.

Please lower your panties/underpant to your knees.
Dr. Carlton: Ngicela wehlile i-panties/ i-underpan ibe semadolweni.

Please could you lie on your left hand side.
Dr. Carlton: Ngicela ulale ngecala lakwa-left.

Please bend your knees closer to your chest.
Dr. Carlton: Ngicela ugobe amadolo uwasondeze esifubeni.

Take deep breaths and relax.
Dr. Carlton: Uphefumulele phezulu bese uya-rileksa.

I am starting.
Dr. Carlton: Sengiyaqala.

Remember to part the buttocks, have a look (skin tags, prolapsed rectal mucosa etc.) before inserting your finger.

If the sphinchter is not relaxed ask the patient to relax it:
Please could you relax.
Dr. Carlton: Ngicela uthambise.
OR
Relax—Thambisa.

If you like the patient to strain, ask them to cough.
Cough.—Khwehlela.

We believe you know what you feeling for in both male and female patients and that you shall discuss and record your findings fully when done.
When done tell the patient that you are taking your finger out, you are done and thank them. Remember to have gauze/ tissue to wipe them afterwards.

I am now coming out.
Dr. Carlton: Sengiyaphuma.

I am done.
Dr. Carlton: Sengiqedile

Thank you.
Dr. Carlton: Ngiyabonga.

Wipe the patient using tissue/gauze.

Proctosigmoidoscopy

Inform the patient about the need of the examination.
Show them the instrument and then prepare it (warming and lubrication).

I am going to use this (show instrument).
Dr. Carlton: Ngizosebenzisa lento.

Ask them to assume the left lateral position (as for anorectal examination previous section).
Then proceed with the procedure. Do not forget to wipe and thank the patients when done.

EXAMINATION FOR HERNIAS

History
Abdominal and groin lumps
Appear / become bigger on straining (e.g. coughing, weightlifting, defecation).
Disappear when lying supine/ termination of the straining activity.

Exposure and positioning

Asking the patient to either lower their underwear or taking them off completely; this shall allow adequate exposure

The standing and laying positions are both useful.

Please lower your panties/underpant to your knees.

Dr. Carlton: Ngicela wehlile i-panties/ i-underpan ibe semadolweni.

Please could you take off your underwear (underpant/ panties).

Dr. Carlton: Ngicela ukhumule i-underwear (i-andapheni/iphenti).

Please could you stand next to the bed?

Dr. Carlton: Ngicela ume eduze kombhede.

Please could you lie on the bed facing up?

Dr. Carlton: Ngiceal ulale embhedeni ubheke phezulu.

To get the patient to strain ask them to cough.

Cough.—Khwehlela.

Male Genitalia

Exposure and positioning

Explain the need for the examination to the patient and what the examination entails.

I would like to examine your front organ.

Dr. Carlton: Ngithanda ukuhlola umphambili.

OR

I would like to examine your private organ.

Dr. Carlton: Ngithanda ukuhlola isitho sangasese.

OR

I would like to examine your penis.

Dr. Carlton: Ngithanda ukuhlola umpipi.

OR

I would like to examine you down there.

Dr. Carlton: Ngithanda ukuhlola ngasezansi.

Ask them to take off their pants

Please could you remove your trouser?

Dr. Carlton: Ngicela ukhumule ibhulukwe.

Please could you lower your underwear?

Dr. Carlton: Ngicela wehlise i-underwear.

OR

Please could you remove your underwear (underpant)?

Dr. Carlton: Ngicela ukhumule i-underwear (i-andapheni).

Please lay on the bed facing up.

Dr. Carlton: Ngicela ulale embhedeni ubheke phezulu.

Please could you open your thighs?

Dr. Carlton: Ngicela uvule amathanga.

Do you have pain?

Dr. Carlton: Bukhona ubuhlungu?

Where? Point?

Dr. Carlton: Kuphi? Khomba.

OR

Tell me when it is painful.
Dr. Carlton: Ungitshele uma kubuhlungu.

And as you continue palpating, ask
Is it painful?
Dr. Carlton: Kubuhlungu?

Female Genitalia

Exposure and Positioning
Privacy and the use of the chaperone are important to attain and maintain especially for male examiners.

I would like to examine your private organ.
Dr. Carlton: Ngithanda ukuhlola isitho sangasese.
OR
I would like to examine you down there.
Dr. Carlton: Ngithanda ukuhlola ngasezansi.
OR
I would like to examine your vigina.
Dr. Carlton: Ngicela ukuhlola indunu.

Ask them to take off their underwear
Dr. Carlton: Ngicela ukhumule i-underwear (iphenti).
OR to lower the underwear to their knees
Dr. Carlton: Ngicela wehlile i-panties ibe semadolweni.

Lie on the bed facing up.
Dr. Carlton: Lala embhedeni ubheke phezulu.

Bend your knees.
Dr. Carlton: Goba amadolo

Open your thighs.
Dr. Carlton: Vula amathanga.

Speculum examination

Explain the need for the examination to the patient and that it shall be uncomfortable tending towards painful.
I would like to examine your private organ using an instrument.

I shall use this instrument (show speculum).
Dr. Carlton: Ngizosebenzila lento.

Preparation is then done, the patient is positioned as required and the procedure proceeds.
You then follow the same positioning procedure as for vaginal examination (previous section). Remember to test the temperature of the speculum on the patient's thigh prior to insertion, it is inhumane to leave out some lubrication and announce entry and retraction of the speculum.

Please open your thighs wider
Dr. Carlton: Vula amathanga kakhulu.

I am about to insert the speculum.
Dr. Carlton: Sengiyasifaka isi-speculum.
Relax
Dr. Carlton: Thambisa

I am now removing it.
Dr. Carlton: Sengiyasikhipha.

EXAMINATION OF THE EXTREMITIES

General

This entails general inspection of the limbs for skin lesions, skeletal abnormalities, trauma, inflammation etc. The important part is to expose to get an adequate view.

The upper body

Take off your upper clothing.
Dr. Carlton: Khumula izingubo zangaphezulu.

Take off your jersey.
Dr. Carlton: Khumule i-jezi
OR
Take off everything.
Dr. Carlton: Khumula konke.

The lower body

Take off your trouser.
Dr. Carlton: Ngicela ukhumule ibhulukwe.

Take off your skirt.
Dr. Carlton: Ngicela ukhumule isiketi.

Take off everything.
Dr. Carlton: Khumula konke.

Remain with your underwear.
Dr. Carlton: Sala nge-underwear.

MUSCULOSKELETAL EXAMINAITON

Most of this part of the examination shall entail demonstrating and observation.
The upper body

The Shoulder Joint

Ask the patient to take off their upper clothing, observe them while they do so and start inspecting (LOOK) the joints (both, the normal and the diseased).

Take off your upper clothing.
Dr. Carlton: Khumula izingubo zangaphezulu.

Remember to observe both sides and compare the two for any unilateral anomalies.
To test and observe winging of the scapula ask the patient to push against the wall.

Push against the wall
Dr. Carlton: Phusha udonga/ubonda.

You can then palpate (FEEL) the joints taking note of pain and the important landmarks also palpate while the patient moves it.

I am going to touch you
Dr. Carlton: Ngizokuthinta.

Tell me if there is pain.
Dr. Carlton: Ungazise uma kubuhlungu.

You then ask the patient to MOVE (active movements) the joints. It is advised that the normal joint is examined first so as to note the limitations of the pathological joint.

Ranges of movement
Abduction:
Lift up your arms above your head (sideways)
Dr. Carlton: Phakamisa izingalo ngaphezu kwekhanda uzise ngasemaceleni.

Abduction and Internal rotation
Ask the patient to touch a point between their scapulae using both the above the head and below the head routes.
Please could you touch between your shoulder-blades with a finger with your arm coming from behind and below?
Dr. Carlton: Ngicela uzithinte eqolo ngaphakathi kweziphanga ingalo iqhamuka ngaphezu kwekhanda uphinde futhi uyiqhamukise ngezansi.

First with one hand then the other.
Dr. Carlton: Yenza ngengalo eyodwa bese wenza ngenye.
OR demonstrate

Do like this (show).

Dr. Carlton: Yenza kanje.

Flexion:

Lift your arms above your head frontwards

Dr. Carlton: Phakamisa izingalo ngaphezu kwekhanda uzise ngaphambili.

OR demonstrate

Do like this (show).

Dr. Carlton: Yenza kanje.

Extension:

Lift your arms from the back (Demonstrate extension).

Dr. Carlton: Phakamiza izingalo uzilule ngemuva.

OR demonstrate

Do like this (show).

Dr. Carlton: Yenza kanje.

Internal and external rotation

(Easier when demonstrated)

Do like this (show).

Dr. Carlton: Yenza kanje.

After this passive range of movement can be tested for

For specialised tests ask the patient to relax while you move them.

Relax.—Thambisa.

OR

Relax—Rileksa (relexer)

The Elbow Joint

Exposure and positioning
Ask the patient to take off their upper clothing (to allow examination of the joint above and the joint below.
Please take off your upper clothing.
Dr. Carlton: Ngicela ukhumule izingubo zangaphezulu.

The patient may be seated or standing.
Sit on the bed/chair.
Dr. Carlton: Hlala embhedeni/esihlalweni.

Remember to look, feel and move.
Both the elbow joints while they are static and while the patient moves them.
Feel the joint for warmth, the joint space, joining bone endings etc.

Flexion:
Flex your arm at the elbow.
Dr. Carlton: Goba ingalo endololwaneni.

Extension:
Extend your arm.
Dr. Carlton: Lula ingalo.

Supination:
Make your palm look upwards.
Dr. Carlton: Bhekisa isanda phezulu.
OR
Dr. Carlton: Khangeza.

Pronation:

Make your palm look downwards.

Dr. Carlton: Bhezisa isandla phansi.

Do like this (show).

Dr. Carlton: Yenza kanje.

Move passive movements for full range of movement.

Relax.

Dr. Carlton: Thambisa.

OR

Dr. Carlton: Relax

For testing strength see neurological examination.

The Wrist and Hand

The LOOK, FEEL & MOVE sequence is followed.

Ask the patient to either take off their upper clothing or pull up their sleeves above the level of the elbow.

Take off your upper clothing.

Dr. Carlton: Khumula izingubo zangaphezulu.

Roll-up your sleeves to above the elbow.

Dr. Carlton: Khuphula imikhono ibe ngaphezu kwendololwane.

Look at the wrist, the palm and fingers for any anomalies.

Touch and feel joint spaces, muscle bulk and areas of tenderness.

Most of the movements shall be demonstrated.
(Flexion, extension, abduction, adduction and other hand movements.)

Do like this (show).
Dr. Carlton: Yenza kanje.

When all the active movements are done passive movements are then done
to complete the examination.
Dr. Carlton: Thambisa.
OR
Dr. Carlton: Relax

The Lower Body
The Hip Joint

Exposure and positioning
For adequate exposure the patient shall remove their lower clothing and
ideally be in their underwear.
You ask them to do just that.

Take off everything.
Dr. Carlton: Khumula konke.
AND
Remain with your underwear.
Dr. Carlton: Sala nge-underwear.

Then the look, feel and move sequence.

Ask the patient to walk and observe their gait to see if it has been affected.
Walk over there (point) and back.
Dr. Carlton: Hamba ujike lapha uphinde ubuye.

The positions of examining this joint are supine and prone positions
Lie on the bed facing up.
Dr. Carlton: Lala embhedeni ubheke phezulu.

Measurements for leg length are done at this point.

Lie on the bed facing down.
Dr. Carlton: Lala embhedeni ubheke phansi.

It is important to remember that hip pain can be referred from elsewhere
(lower back) or be referred to other places (e.g. knee)

For active movements
Abduction:
Open your thighs.
Dr. Carlton: Vula amathanga
This can also be done against resistance.

Adduction:
With open thighs,
Close your thighs.—Vala amathanga
OR
From a neutral position,
Cross your legs.—Phambanisa izinyawo.
This can also be done against resistance.

Flexion:

Lift your leg straight up.

Dr. Carlton: Phakamise umlenze uwuqondisile.

To determine if the source of the leg length descrepency (above or below the knee), ask the patient to bend their knees and make out your dimensions. Bend your knees.

Dr. Carlton: Goba amadolo.

Extension (done on prone position or against resistance on a hip that was previously flexed)

On a prone position,

Please could you lift your leg up backwards?

Dr. Carlton: Ngicela uphakamise unyawo ulise emuva.

Or

On supine position, passively lift the lower limb then ask

Put your foot down.

Dr. Carlton: Beka unyawo phansi.

Rotations: it is important to remember which one is done during an examination with a flexed and an extended knee. Both examinations i.e. with the hip and knee flexed to 90 degrees are given as examples here. The examination done with a flexed knee allows measurement of the angulation of rotation and is for that reason better than the straight leg examination. These are normaly done as passive movements.

Internal Rotation:

Flexed hip and knee [done passively]:

Dr. Carlton: Thambisa.

OR

Dr. Carlton: Relax

On a supine patient, with the hip and knee bent to 90 degrees, foot in the air ask:

Please move your foot outwards/this side (point direction).

Dr. Carlton: Yisa unyawo ngaphandle/ngapha.

Straight leg:

Move your foot inwards/this side (point direction).

Dr. Carlton: Yisa unyawo ngaphakathi/ngapha.

External Rotation

Flexed knee:

Move your foot inwards/this side (point direction).

Dr. Carlton: Yisa unyawo ngaphakathi/ngapha.

Straight leg:

Move your foot outwards/this side (point direction).

Dr. Carlton: Yisa unyawo ngaphandle/ngapha.

For passive movements and special tests (e.g. FABER i.e. hip Flexion, Abduction and External Rotation) ask the patient to relax and then move the joint noting pain, range of motion and resistance to movement.

Dr. Carlton: Thambisa.

OR

Dr. Carlton: Relax

The Knee Joint

Exposure and Positioning

Ask the patient to take off their lower clothing; a gown and underwear are ideal for complete examination.
Take off everything below the waist.
Dr. Carlton: Khumula konke ngaphansi kokhalo.

Remain with your underwear.
Dr. Carlton: Sala nge-underwear.

Ask them to walk in your rooms if you did not see them walk in or you are aiming to observe any changes in gait.
Walk over there and back.
Dr. Carlton: Hamba ujike lapha uphinde ubuye.

Remember to examine the joint above and below for completeness.

Look
Look at both the knees for symmetry, scars, muscle wasting, inflammation, deformities etc. and compare.

Feel
Feel both knees for warmth; ask about pain, joint space, ends of articulating bones. Examples of questions you can ask about a certain anomaly e.g. an unusual discoloration around the knee

What is this?
Dr. Carlton: Yini le?

Khekheleza: Ibala

Were you injured?
Dr. Carlton: Walimala?
Khekheleza: Hhe eeh.

Is it painful?
Dr. Carlton: Ibuhlungu
Khekheleza: Hhaai

What caused it?
Dr. Carlton: Yadalwa yini?
Khekheleza: Angazi.

When?
Dr. Carlton: Nini?
Khekheleza: Ngazalwa nayo.

Move.
For active movements ask the patient to:
Flexion:
Bend your knee.
Dr. Carlton: Goba idolo.

Extension:
Extend your knee.
Dr. Carlton: Lula idolo
For passive movements ask the patient to relax the joint and you shall move it.
Dr. Carlton: Thambisa.
OR

Dr. Carlton: Relax

Also ask the patient to relax their joints to be able to carry out special tests.

The Ankle joint and small joints of the foot

Exposure and positioning

The shoes and socks must be removed; the leg exposed up to above the level of the knee. Taking a look at the shoes may give some clues.

Remove your shoes and socks.
Dr. Carlton: Khumula izicathulo namasokisi.

Roll up your trouser to the knee.
Dr. Carlton: Phakamisa ibhulukwe ulibeke phezu kwamadolo.

Pull up your skirt to the knee
Dr. Carlton: Phakamisa isiketi sibe semadolweni.

Remove your trouser.
Dr. Carlton: Khumula ibhulukwe.

Observing the gait is crucial; to see joint pathology and if it has been affected by it.
Walk over there and back?
Dr. Carlton: Hamba ujike lapha uphinde ubuye.

Walk on your toes.
Dr. Carlton: Hamba ngezinzwane.
OR

Dr. Carlton: Hamba ucokeme

The seated, standing and laying positions are to be used for the examination. Having the the foot and leg of the patient on your lap is the perfect position for comprehensive examination.

Sit on the chair/ bed.

Dr. Carlton: Hlala esitulweni/embhedeni.

Lie on the bed facing up.—Lala embhedeni ubheke phezulu.

Remember to look, feel and move.

For active movements

Plantar Flexion:

Bend your foot downwards.—Gobisa unyawo luye phansi.

OR

(Demonstrate with hands)

Bend your foot like this.

Dr. Carlton: Goba unyawo kanje.

Plantar Extension:

Bend your foot upwards.

Dr. Carlton: Gobisa unyawo luye phezulu.

OR

(Demonstrate with hands)

Bend your foot like this

Dr. Carlton: Goba unyawo kanje.

For the toes

Bend your toes downwards.

Dr. Carlton: Yisa izinzwane phansi.

Bend your toes upwards.
Dr. Carlton: Yisa izinzwane phezulu.
(Demonstrate with hands)

The other movements may have to be demonstrated (inversion and eversion.)
Inversion:
Turn your foot inward.
(Demonstrate)
Dr. Carlton: Jikisa unyawo ulise ngaphakathi.

Eversion:
Turn your foot outward.
Dr. Carlton: Jikisa unyawo ulise ngaphandle.

For passive movements ask the patient to relax their joints and you shall move them.
Dr. Carlton: Thambisa.
OR
Dr. Carlton: Relax

NEUROLOGICAL

Focused History:
This part of the examination should be done routinely.
The higher neurological functions and mental status examination are beyond the scope of the manual as particular understanding of the language

is a prerequisite. However inappropriate behaviour and other apparent "unusual" observations should be noted.

It may be a suggestion on history or other examination that there is a neurological deficit. Other deeply specific neurological examinations (testing for dysphasia type) may prove to be impossible to carry out and are beyond the scope of this manual.

The general and systematic examination shall be done appropriately prior to examing the neurological system. The neurological examination is done in different fashions depending on the history and timeoulsy it not completed. In this manual the format of examining cranial nerves sequentially, the tone, power, sensation and cerebeller functions shall be used.

EXAMINATION OF THE CRAINIAL NERVES

CRANIAL NERVE I

Focused History:
This will involve the loss of or reduced sense of smell and taste. It may also be trauma to the cribriform plate and nasal cerebrospinal fluid leaks.

Examination:
I would like to know if you can identify substances throught smelling them.
Dr. Carlton: Ngithanda ukwazi ukuthi ungakhona ukusho ukuthi uhogela ini ngaphandle kokuyibona.

Please close your eyes?
Dr. Carlton: (Ngiyakucela). Vala amehlo.

Do not peep through.
Dr. Carlton: Ungalunguzi.

Close one nostril with your finger.
Dr. Carlton: Vala ikhala elilodwa ngomunwe.

One nostril is done then the other.
Pepper.—Upelepele.
Coffee.—Ikhofi.
Cinnamon. (likely not to be known)—I-sinamoni.
Perfume.—I-perfume.
Ammonia—i-ammonia (also likely not to be known and not a good substance to use anyway.

CRANIAL NERVE II:

Focused History:
Mono-(bi-)ocular blindness, suspected glaucoma, risk factors for retinal disease (diabetes, hypertension), trauma etc

EXAMINATION
Visual fields
I am going to sit in front of you.
Dr. Carlton: Ngizohlala phambi kwakho.

Cover your one eye (left/right) with your hand.
Dr. Carlton: Vala ihlo lakho lakwa—(left/right).

To demonstrate
Do like this (show).—Yenza kanje.

Look into my eye with the other eye.
Dr. Carlton: Bheka ehlweni lami ngelinye ihlo lakho.

Do not turn your head or your eye.
Dr. Carlton: Ungalijikisi ikhanda noma ihlo.

Let me know (say yes) when you can see this object (show object).
Dr. Carlton: Ungazise uma ubona le nto. (uthi yebo)

The eyes are then done in succession, while defects in the visual fields are noted.

To proceed to examining the other eye
We are now going to do the other eye.
Dr. Carlton: Sezizokwenze leli elinye ihlo.

Visual Acuity
Please tell me the letters on the chart in succession.
Dr. Carlton: (Ngiyakucela). Isho amagama ezinhlamvu eziseshadini ngokulandelana kwazo.

Please say to which direction the prongs of the 3/M/W/E are facing (for the E chart).
Dr. Carlton: Isho ukuthi izimfologo zohlamvu zibheke ngakuphi.

Here you may have to inform the patient about the E being a trident and practice showing them the different direction e.g. in M the trindent is facing down, in 3 the trident is facing the left etc. Thereafter you may proceed to the E chart.

Please name the letter that is pointed at.
Dr. Carlton: Isho igama lohlamvu elizokhonjiwa.

What letter is this (while pointing at different letters)

Dr. Carlton: Ubani lo.

Ophthalmoscopy
I would like to look at your eye. (with the instrument [show])
Dr. Carlton: Ngithanda ukukubheka ehlweni.

I shall not be painful.
Dr. Carlton: Angeke kube buhlungu.

It is just bright light
Dr. Carlton: Ukukhanya okuxhophayo

I shall get really close to you.
Dr. Carlton: Ngizosondela eduze kakhulu.

Please look straight ahead.
Dr. Carlton: Bheka phambili.

Do not look at the light.
Dr. Carlton: Ungabheki ukukhanya.

If there is an object to focus on ask the patient to look at that e.g. focus on the red dot.
Dr. Carlton: Bheka indilinga ebomvu.

You then proceed with opthalmoscopy.

If finding the macula is challenging ask the patient to look at the light.
Look at the light
Dr. Carlton: Bheka ukukhanya

CRANIAL NERVE III, IV & VI

Focused History:

Do you see double?

Dr. Carlton: Ingabe ubona izinto zizimbili?

Khekheleza: Yebo, ngibona ngambili

Do you find it difficult to read?

Dr. Carlton: Ukuthola kunzima ukufunda?

Do you find it difficult to look to the right/ left?

Dr. Carlton: Ukuthola kunzima ukubheka kwa-right/left?

Khekheleza: Kunzima ukubheka kwa-left.

Does one of your eyes look at one place all the time?

Dr. Carlton: Ingabe ihlo lakho elilodwa lihlala libheke endaweni eyodwa?

Khekheleza: ihlo lakwa-left lihlala libheke kwa-right.

Other systemic disease like autoimmune hyperthyroidism, neurological deficits may warrant examination of this group of cranial nerves.
Testing for nystagmus is also done at this point.

EXAMINATION:

Follow this object (show object)/ my finger with your eyes.

Dr. Carlton: Landela lento (show object)/ umunwe wami ngamehlo.

Do not turn your head.

Dr. Carlton: Ungaliphendulu ikhanda lakho.

CRANIAL NERVE V

Focused History:

Be weary of herpes zoster pain, trigeminal neuralgia, sinusitis and teeth root pain as part of the complaint.

Do you have decreased or no sensation on parts of the face?

Dr. Carlton: Ingabe kukhona lapho ungezwa khona uma uthintwa ebusweni?

Khekheleza: Izihlathi zami zindikindiki.

Numb—Ndikindiki

Do you have jaw weakness?

Dr. Carlton: Ingabe unobuthakathaka bomhlathi?

Khekheleza: Yebo, kunzima ukuhlafuna inyama

Do you have difficulties speaking?

Dr. Carlton: Unayo inkinga ngokukhuluma?

Khekheleza: Yebo angikhoni ukumemeza

Do you have pain on your teeth or their roots?

Dr. Carlton: Unabo ubuhlungu emazinyweni noma ezimpandeni zawo?

Khekheleza: Yebo, ngihlushwa izinyo elibolile.

Do you have pain in your eyes?

Dr. Carlton: Unabo ubuhlungu bamehlo?

Khekheleza: Yebo, seloku ngagwazeka ehlweni ihlo linokuba buhlungu.

Examination

Find a place with intact sensation (e.g. area of a forearm) and test the sensory stimulus there.

Light touch
Can you feel this touching you?
Dr. Carlton: Uyayizwa lento ekuthintayo?
Khekheleza: Yebo,

Response: the expected response is yes for all the questions on the chosen site of normal sensation.

Can you feel this pricking you?
Dr. Carlton: Uyayizwa lento ekuhlabayo?
Khekheleza: Yebo,

Can you feel this burning you?
Dr. Carlton: Uyayizwa lento ekushisayo?
Khekheleza: Yebo,

Then ask the patient to close their eyes and do the same on the face. Remember to be gentle.

Close your eyes.
Dr. Carlton: Vala amehlo.

Say yes if you can feel a touch/prick/burn on your face.
Dr. Carlton: Uthi yebo uma uzwa ikuthinta/ikuhlaba/ikushisa ebusweni.
OR
Better yet ask the patient if what they feel?
What do you feel?
Dr. Carlton: Uzwa ini?

Touch—Ukuthinta
Prick—Ukuhlaba
Warm—Ukushisa
Cold—Ukubanda
Vibrate—Ukuzamazama

CRANIAL NERVE VII

Focused History
Muscle palsies?
Have you noticed any changes on your facial appearance?
Dr. Carlton: Uke waxwaya ushintsho endleleni ubuso bakho obubukeka ngayo?
Khekheleza: Yebo,

If the response is yes and the explanation is not volunteered ask for it.
Please explain.
Dr. Carlton: Ngicela uchaze.
Khekheleza: Angikhoni ukuvala ihlo lakwa-left.

Can you move both sides of your face?
Dr. Carlton: Uyakhona ukunyakazisa izinxenye zobuso bakho kanye kanye.
Khekheleza: Ubuso ngapha (pointing to the right with the left finger) abusebenzi.

Have you noticed you eye closing by itself?
Dr. Carlton: Kuyenzeka ihlo lakho lizivalekele?
Khekheleza: Cha

EXAMINATION

Please look up without moving your head. (to see forehead creases)
Dr. Carlton: Ngicela ubheke phezulu ungalinyakazisi ikhanda.

Close your eyes tightly.
Dr. Carlton: Vala amehlo uwaqinise.

Do not allow me to open them.
Dr. Carlton: Ungangivumeli ukuthi ngiwavule.

Please blow your cheeks (may have to demonstrate).
Dr. Carlton: Futha izihlathi.

Do not let the air out when I press on the cheeks.
Dr. Carlton: Ungawukhiphi umoya uma ngikucindezela ezihlathini.

Show your teeth.
Dr. Carlton: Veza amazinyo.
OR
Smile.
Dr. Carlton: Sineka.

Close your moth tightly.
Dr. Carlton: Vala umlomo uwuqinise.
Do not let me open it.
Dr. Carlton: Ungavumi ngiwuvule.

CRANIAL NERVE VIII

Focused History:

Do you have problems hearing?

Dr. Carlton: Unenkinga nokuzwa ngezindlebe?

Khekheleza: Indlebe yami yakwa left ayizwa kahle.

If the response is yes and the explanation is not volunteered ask for it.

Please explain.

Dr. Carlton: Ngicela uchaze.

Khekheleza: Noma umsindo ungakhona ngiwuzwa kahle kwa-right.

Do you hear better with your right or left ear?

Dr. Carlton: Uzwa kangcono (better) ngendlebe yakwa-right noma yakwa-left?

Khekheleza: Kwa-right

Do you have ringing in your ears?

Dr. Carlton: Kukhona umsindo onsininizayo owuzwayo?

Khekheleza: Cha.

Do you hear any unusual sounds in your ears?

Dr. Carlton: Ikhona imsindo engajwayelekile oyizwayo?

Khekheleza: Cha

Are you feeling dizzy?

Dr. Carlton: Sikuphethe isiyezi?

Khekheleza: Cha

Dou you feel like you are moving when you are not?

Dr. Carlton: Uke uzizwe ngathi uyanyakaza kepha unganyakazi

Khekheleza: Yebo, uma ngiphethwe isiyezi

Do you see the world spinning?

Dr. Carlton: Ubona umhlaba ujikeleza?

Khekheleza: Cha

EXAMINATION

These examinations should be done with the eyes closed.

Close your eyes.

Dr. Carlton: Vala amehlo.

The ticking clock test (the clock is moved closer to the patient's ear from a further position.)

Please tell me when you start hearing the ticking of the clock.

Dr. Carlton: Ngicela ungazise uma uqala ukuzwa umsindo wezingalo zewashi.

Khekheleza: OK

The finger rubbing or any other sound (rubbing the palmar surface of the index finger on that of the thumb).

Please can you tell me if you can hear any sound?

Dr. Carlton: Ngitshele uma kukhona umsindo owuzwayo?

Khekheleza: Ngiyawuzwa

What is the sound?

Dr. Carlton: Umsindo wani?

Khekheleza: Iminwe yakho ihlikihlana.

When the testing is complete.

Open your eyes.

Dr. Carlton: Vula amehlo.

THE RHINE'S TEST

I am going to hold this fork in front of your ear and also put it behind your ear.

Dr. Carlton: Ngizobamba le mfologo ngaphimbi kwendlebe yakho ngiphinde ngiyibeke ngemuva kwendlebe.

Tell me where you hear it the loudest. In front or behind the ear?

Dr. Carlton: Ngazise ukuthi umsindo omkhulu uwuzwa ngakuphi. Ngaphambili noma ngemuva kwendlebe?

Khekheleza: Ngaphambili.

WEBER'S TEST

I am going to put this fork on the top of your head.

Dr. Carlton: Ngizobeka le mfologo phezulu ekhanda.

On the forehead—Esiphongweni

On the chin—Esilevini

On your lower teeth—Emazinyweni akho engezansi.

Please tell me on which side you hear it better. Right or left hand side?

Dr. Carlton: Ngazise ukuthi uyizwa kakhulu ngakuphi. Kwa-right noma kwa-left.

Khekheleza: Right/left (which is an abnormal finding)

Khekheleza: Kuyalingana ezindlebeni zombili.

CRANIAL NERVE IX

Focused History

Do you have problems swallowing food?

Dr. Carlton: Unazo izinkiga nokugwinya ukudla?

Khekheleza: Yebo, kuyangibamba ukudla uma komile.

Do you have problems swallowing water?

Dr. Carlton: Unazo izinkinga nokugwinya amanzi?

Khekheleza: Yebo, aphuma ngamakhala.

Do you have an unusual sensation on the ears when chewing food?

Dr. Carlton: Kuyenzeka ube nemizwa engajwayelekile ezindlebeni uma uhlafuna ukudla?

Khekheleza: Yebo

EXAMINATION

Listen closely to speech to assess the hoarseness of the voice.

You can ask the patient to repeat expressions if required.

Say "Noddy is a naughty boy".

Dr. Carlton: Ithi "Noddy is a naughty boy"

Khekheleza: Noddy is a naughty boy

Listen to the character of the cough.

Please cough.

Dr. Carlton: Khwehlela.

Khekheleza: "Coughs"

The gag reflex

I would like to look into your mouth, open your mouth and stick out your tongue.
Dr. Carlton: Ngicela ukubona emlonyeni, vula umlomo ukhiphe ulimi.

I shall depress your tongue with the spatula and touch your throat.
Dr. Carlton: Ngizokwehlisa ulimi nge-spatula bese ngithinta umphimbo.

To see the deviations of the uvula
Please say "aah"/ "eeh".
Dr. Carlton: Ithi "aah" / "eeh"
OR
Dr. Carlton: Thani "aah" / "eeh"
Khekheleza: "aah" / "eeh"

The water regurgitation test
Please drink this glass of water as fast as you can.
Dr. Carlton: Ngicela uphuze lamanzi uphangise uma ukhona.
Khekheleza: OK (then drinks the water offered).

CRANIAL NERVE X

Focused History
These questions are non-specific.
Do you feel light-headed on standing up?
Dr. Carlton: Uphathwa isiyezi uma usukuma?
Khekheleza: Cha

Do you ever feel your heart beating too fast or too slow?

Dr. Carlton: Uke uzwe inhliziyo ishaya nokushesha noma ishayela phansi?

Khekheleza: Nginokuyizwa ishaya kancane.

Examination is done together with that of the nineth cranial nerve.

CRANIAL NERVE XI

Focused History:

Do you have problems with turning your head?

Dr. Carlton: Uba nenkinga uma uphendula ikhanda?

Khekheleza: Cha, ngaphandle-nje uma kukhathele intamo.

Torticollis

Do you have a muscular problem that makes your head look on only one direction?

Dr. Carlton: Ingabe unenkinga eyenza ukuthi ikhanda lihlale libheke engxenyeni eyodwa?

Khekheleza: Cha

The "I don't know sign"

Do you have problems with lifting your shoulders?

Dr. Carlton: Kukhona inkinga uma uphakamisa amahlombe?

Khekheleza: Cha

EXAMINAITON

Turn your head to the left then to the right.

Dr. Carlton: Phendula ikhanda ubheke kwa-left bese ubheka kwa-right.

Lift your shoulders (the "I don't know" sign).
Dr. Carlton: Phakamisa amahlombe.

You may have to demonstrate.
Say: Do like this. [Shrug].
Dr. Carlton: Yenza kanje.

Lift your soulders while I push them down.
Dr. Carlton: Phakamisa amahlombe mina ngizowaphushela phansi.

Look to the right, and then turn your head to the left against my hand.
Dr. Carlton: Bheka kwa-right bese ubheka kwa-left ungavumi ngikubhekise ngakwa-right.

Look to the left, and then turn your head to the right against my hand.
Bheka kwa-left, bese ubhekwa kwa-right ungavumi ngikubhekise kwa-left.

CRANIAL NERVE XII (HYPOGOSSAL NERVE)

HISTORY
Do you have problems swallowing food?
Dr. Carlton: Unayo inkinga nokugwinya ukudla?
Khekheleza: Yebo uma ngigwinya okuningi kuyangibamba.

Do you ever choke on your tongue?
Dr. Carlton: Kujenzeka uxhilwe ulimi lwakho?
Khekheleza: Cha

Do you have trouble with saying words correctly?
Dr. Carlton: Unayo inkinga nokusho amagama kahle?
Khekheleza: Yebo, ngiyathefuza
OR
Khekheleza: Yebo, ngiyathefuya.

EXAMINATION
I would like to look in your mouth.
Dr. Carlton: Ngithanda ukubona emlonyeni wakho.

Open your mouth.
Dr. Carlton: Vula umlomo.

Stick out your tongue.
Dr. Carlton: Khipha ulimi.

Move your tongue up.
Dr. Carlton: Yisa ulimi phezulu.

Down—phansi
To the right—kwa-right
To the left—kwa-left

Alternatively you can point directions
Move it to this side
Dr. Carlton: Luyise ngapha
Then to this side—Nangapha.

SENSORY EVALUATION AND EXAMINATION

Most parts of this examination are carried out with the patients' eyes closed. One needs to firstly find a place where the patient has normal sensation and use this to test the stimulus to be applied.

It is important to have all the instruments needed e.g. tuning fork, to explain to the patient on what is to be done and not to cause harm to the patients (e.g. using the same pin for different patients/ applying too much pressure)

To evaluate the stimulus applied ask if the patient can fee the different stimuli.

Do you feel this touching you?

Dr. Carlton: Uyezwa ukuthi ngiyakuthinta lapha?

Khekheleza: Yebo

(Should be a yes if you are touching the body part with normal sensation)

With a sharp point of the pin
Pricking
Do you feel this pricking you?

Dr. Carlton: Uyezwa ukuthi ngiyakuhlaba lapha?

OR
Stabbing
Dr. Carlton: Ukugwaza

With a warm object
Warming
Dr. Carlton: Ukushisa

With a cool object
Cooling—ukubandisa

With a vibrating tuning fork
Vibration—ukuzamazama

May use different objects to also check if the patient understands, in which case you ask what the patient feels.
What do you feel now?
Dr. Carlton: Uzwa ini manje?
Khekheleza: Ukuzamazama

The patient should be told that they are going to close their eyes and say if they can feel/ distinguish between the different stimuli.

I am going to touch you with cotton wool; say yes if you feel me toucing you.
Dr. Carlton: Ngizokuthinta nge-cotton wool uthi yebo uma uzwa ngikuthinta.
Say yes if you can feel me touching you.
Dr. Carlton: Uthi-yes uma uzwa ngikuthinta.
Khekheleza: OK

Alternatively you can ask patients to tell you what it is they feel on the particular part of the body and whether it is the left side or the right.

What do you feel?
Dr. Carlton: Uzwa ini manje?

Is it on the right or left hand side?

Dr. Carlton: Kwa-right noma kwa-left.

OR

On which side?

Dr. Carlton: Ngakuphi?

Khekheleza: Kwa-left (as appropriate)

Close your eyes.

Dr. Carlton: Vala amehlo.

Open your eyes.

Dr. Carlton: Vula amehlo.

The primary senses of touch, pain and vibration should be tested for. For completenes temperature, pressure and the different modes of touch need to be evaluated as well.

It is imperative to evaluate intensity.

Does it feel the same as on the area of normal sensation (e.g. face, arm etc)

Dr. Carlton: Kuzwakala kufana kunasebusweni/engalweni?

Alternatively you can point

Is it the same as here (point)?

Dr. Carlton: Kuyafana nalapha (point)?

MOTOR EVALUATION

This element of the examination includes observation, inspection, palpation, muscle tone testing, functional testing and strength of different muscle groups.

Exposure and positioning

The patient has to be adequately exposed for the observation and inspection parts of the examination. Muscle bulk, fasciculation, abnormal posture, twitches etc. need to be looked out for. Ask the patient to take off their clothing and remain in their underwear/ sequentially examine the upper then the lower body.

Take off everything.

Dr. Carlton: Khumula konke.

Remain with your underwear.

Dr. Carlton: Sala nge-underwear.

Muscle tone testing

Ask the patient to relax and you shall move their joints. Remember to move the joint through its full range of motion at least twice (and not more than 5 times) at different paces.

Relax and let me move your joints.

Dr. Carlton: Thambisa bese uyekela mina ngikunyakazise.

Relax.

Dr. Carlton: Thambisa.

OR

Relax

Dr. Carlton: Relaxer

Power

Muscle testing and strength test.

Remember to grade the power of muscle group examined. Ask the patient to firstly move the joint unopposed and then you may apply resistance.

The upper limb
Shoulder joint
Lift up your arms above your head (sideways)
Dr. Carlton: Phakamisa izingalo ngaphezu kwekhanda uzise ngasemaceleni.

Do like this (show).
Dr. Carlton: Yenza kanje.
The action can then be done against resistance.

Elbow joint

Flex your arm at the elbow.
Dr. Carlton: Goba ingalo endololwaneni.
The action can then be done against resistance.

Extend your arm.
Dr. Carlton: Lula ingalo.
The action can then be done against resistance.

Supination:
Make your palm look upwards.
Dr. Carlton: Bhekisa isanda phezulu.
OR
Dr. Carlton: Khangeza.

Pronation:
Make your palm look downwards.
Dr. Carlton: Bhezisa isandla phansi.

Wrist and hand

Make a fist.

Dr. Carlton: Fumba isibhakela/inqindi.

Do like this (show).

Dr. Carlton: Yenza kanje.

Do not let me open your hand.

Dr. Carlton: Ungavumi ngikuvule isandla.

Other movements shall then be demonstrated, let the patient know that they are to maintain the assumed action against your resistance.

Do like this (show).

Dr. Carlton: Yenza kanje.

Keep it like that

Dr. Carlton: Umise kanjalo.

Do not allow me to turn it/break it.

Dr. Carlton: Ungavumi ngikujikise/ngikuyekise

Lower Limb.

Please could you walk over there (point) and back.

Dr. Carlton: Ngicela uhambe ujike lapha uphinde ubuye.

Hip Joint

The positions of examining this joint are supine and prone positions

Please lie on the bed facing up.

Dr. Carlton: Ngicela ulale embhedeni ubheke phezulu.

Please lie on the bed facing down.

Dr. Carlton: Ngicela ulale embhedeni ubheke phansi.

Abduction:

Open your thighs.

Dr. Carlton: Vula amathanga

This can also be done against resistance.

Adduction:

With open thighs,

Close your thighs.

Dr. Carlton: Vala amathanga

OR

From a neutral position,

Cross your legs.

Dr. Carlton: Phambanisa izinyawo.

This can also be done against resistance.

Flexion:

Lift your leg straight up.

Dr. Carlton: Phakamise unyawo uluqondisile.

Extension (done on prone position or against resistance on a hip that was previously flexed)

On a prone position,

Please could you lift your leg up backwards.

Dr. Carlton: Ngicela uphakamise unyawo ulise emuva.

Or

On supine position, passively lift the lower limb then ask

Put your foot down.

Dr. Carlton: Beka unyawo phansi.

Knee Joint
Bend your knee.
Dr. Carlton: Goba idolo.
The action can then be done against resistance.

Extend your knee.
Dr. Carlton: Lula idolo
The action can then be done against resistance.

Ankle and foot
Walk on your toes.
Dr. Carlton: Hamba ngezinzwane.
OR Hamba ucokeme

The movements on these joints are easily done by demonstration with the hands asking the patient to do the movement with their feet.
For strength and resistance testing you ask the patient to sustain the assumed position while you apply resistance or repeat the action against resistance.

Do like this (show).
Dr. Carlton: Yenza kanje.

Hold that position and do not let me break it.
Dr. Carlton: Yima kanjalo ungavumi ngikujikise.

Do it again (apply resistance at this point).
Dr. Carlton: Yenza futhi OR Phinda
Again.
Dr. Carlton: Futhi.

Toes

Bend your toes.

Dr. Carlton: Goba izinzwane.

Extend your toes.

Dr. Carlton: Lula izinzwane.

Or demonstrate movements with your hands.

Do like this (show).

Dr. Carlton: Yenza kanje.

Hold that position and do not let me break it.

Dr. Carlton: Yima kanjalo ungavumi ngikujikise.

Do it again (apply resistance at this point).

Dr. Carlton: Yenza futhi.

Again.

Dr. Carlton: Futhi.

Reflexes

You need to ask the patient to assume the desired position and relax. You shall then move the joint to the position of your choice and elicit the reflexes.

Lie on the bed facing up.

Dr. Carlton: Lala embhedeni ubheke phezulu.

Sit up.

Dr. Carlton: Vuka uhlale

Sit on the bed.
Dr. Carlton: Hlala embhedeni

Relax.
Dr. Carlton: Thambisa.
OR
Relax
Dr. Carlton: Relaxer

Plantar Reflex
Inform the patient about your proceedings.
I am going to scrape under your foot with this (show instrument).
Dr. Carlton: Ngizokuhwaya onyaweni ngalento (show instrument).

Cerebella Functions

Vertigo—discussed as part of the history

Nystagmus—ask the patint to look at an object without turning their heads.
Move this to the lateral extremes and observe for presence of nystagmus.
Follow this with your eyes (show object).
Dr. Carlton: Landela lento ngamehlo.

Do not turn your head.
Dr. Carlton: Ungalijikisi ikhanda.

Dysmitria—Past pointing
Ask the patient to do a rapid movement which they shall stop abruptly.
You may have to demonstrate.

Lift your arms quickly and stop at shoulder level.

Dr. Carlton: Phakamisa izingalo masisha bese uzimise uma seziqondene namahlombe.

Do like this (Demonstrate)

Dr. Carlton: Yenza kanje.

The other components are either observed or covered by the following examinations.

Finger-nose testing

a. With the patient seated, position your index finger at a point in space in front of the patient.

b. Instruct the patient to move their index finger between your finger and their nose.

Touch your nose with your finger and then touch my finger. Like this (demonstrate).

Dr. Carlton: Thinta ikhala lakho ngomunwe bese uthinta umunwe wami. Reposition your finger after each touch.

c. Then test the other hand.

d. Do it with this hand as well. (Point hand)

Dr. Carlton: Yenza nangalesi isandla.

Rapid alternating finger movements

    a. Ask the patient to touch the tips of each finger to the thumb of the same hand.
    b. Test both hands.

Do like this. (do the finger-thumb walking).

Dr. Carlton: Yenza kanje.

Do it with this hand as well. (point hand)

Dr. Carlton: Yenza nangalesi isandla.
OR
Rapid alternating hand movements
Direct the patient to touch first the palm and then the dorsal side of one hand repeatedly against their thigh.

    a. Then test the other hand.

It is easier when demonstrated.
Do like this (Demonstrate).
Dr. Carlton: Yenza kanje.
Heel to shin testing
The patient has to be supine for this examination.
Direct the patient to move the heel of one foot up and down along the top of the other shin.

Slide your heel on your shin, first down then up.

Dr. Carlton: Hambisa isithende embaleni, usise ezansi bese usisa phezulu.

Then test the other foot.

Dr. Carlton: Bese wenza nomunye umlenze.

Gait Testing

Walk over there (point) and back.

Dr. Carlton: Hamba ujike lapha uphinde ubuye.

SITUATIONS

ASKING THE PATIENT to come in.
Dr. Carlton: Ngicela ungene.

OR

Dr. Carlton: (Ngiyakuela). Ngena

OR

Dr. Carlton: Owokuqala

Outpatients' clinic (calling the next patient)

Next person
Dr. Carlton: Olandelayo.

PROCEDURES

TAKING BLOOD SPECIMENS
Greet the patient if you have not.
Introduce yourself.
May I take blood for some tests? (blood cell amounts, kidney function, ion, liver function, infection, HIV, and so on)

Dr. Carlton: Ngicela ukuthatha igazi lizohlolwa.
Khekheleza: Uhlola ini?

(amandla egazi, ukusebenza kwezinso, ukusebenza kwesibindi, izinhlamvu zotswayi, amagciwane, i-HIV, kanjalo kanjalo)

I am goint to prick/inject you on the arm.
Dr. Carlton: Ngizokuhlaba/jova engalweni.

Arm—ingalo
On the arm—engalweni

Groin—enqulu
On the groin—enqulwini

Neck—intamo
On the neck—entanyeni

Leg—unyawo
On the leg—onyaweni /enyaweni

Giving injections
Greet the patient if you have not.
Introduce yourself.
I am here to give you an injection.
Dr. Carlton: Ngilapha ukuzokujova.

I am going to inject on your bum.
Dr. Carlton: Ngizokujova esinqeni.

On the shoulder—ehlombe
On the arm—engalweni

On the thigh—ethangeni

Putting up a drip
Greet the patient if you have not.
Introduce yourself.
May I put up a drip to give you fluids?
Dr. Carlton: Ngicela ukufaka i-drip yamanzi.

Blood—igazi

I am going to prick you on the arm.
Dr. Carlton: Ngizokuhlaba/jova engalweni

Doing a lumber puncture
In the interest of ease while conducting this procedure patient cooperation
is essential; ensure that they have all the instructions and follow them.

Greet the patient if you have not.
Introduce yourself.
I have to get fluid/water from your back for tests.
Dr. Carlton: Kumele ngithole uketshezi/amanzi eqolo luzohlolwa.

It is going to be painful.
Dr. Carlton: Kuzoba buhlungu.

But you must be strong as this test is important.
Dr. Carlton: Kodwa kumele uqinisele ngoba lohlolo lubalulekile.

I am going to prick you on your back/on your spine.
Dr. Carlton: Ngizokuhlaba eqolo/emgogodleni.

You then give instructions sequentially:

Bend your back.
Dr. Carlton: Goba iqolo.

Put your chin on your chest.
Dr. Carlton: Beka isilevu esifubeni.

Fold your arms on your chests.
Dr. Carlton: Songa izandla esifubeni.

Do not jump.
Dr. Carlton: Ungagxumi.

Be brave and strong.
Dr. Carlton: Qinisela.

Hang in there.
Dr. Carlton: Bekezela.

REFERENCES

1. http://www.meded.ucsd.edu/clinicalmed. Accessed 4 September 2007.
2. *http://www.southafrica.info/about/people/language.htm. Accessed February 15th 2010.*
3. http://www.IsiZulu.net. Zulu-English dictionary. Accessed on 19 Febuary 2010
4. N. J. Talley, S. O'Connor. Clinical examinations. A Systematic Guide to Physical Examination. 5Th Edition. Churchill Livingston Elsevier, 2006.

INDEX

A

D

E

F

G

I

J

K

L

M

N

O

P

W